Spilled Coffee

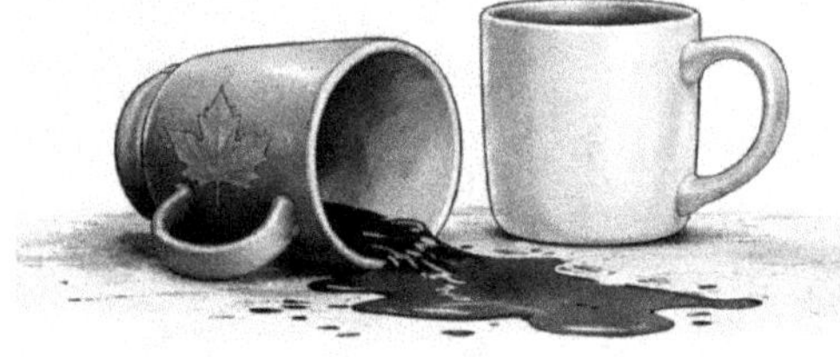

Spilled Coffee

J.D. Roff

Liminal Ground Literary Press

Spilled Coffee

Copyright © 2026 by J.D. Roff

All rights reserved. No part of this book may be reproduced, stored in a retrieval system, or transmitted in any form or by any means—electronic, mechanical, photocopying, recording, or otherwise—without the prior written permission of the publisher, except for brief quotations used in reviews or scholarly works.

Published by
Liminal Ground Literary Press

ISBN: 978-1-972520-01-7

This is a work of fiction. Names, characters, places, and incidents are either products of the author's imagination or are used fictitiously. Any resemblance to actual persons, living or dead, events, or locales is entirely coincidental.

First edition

Printed in the United States of America

To my Rock Steady Boxing family and the coaches who saw our strength when we couldn't see it.

A Word About This Book

You're holding a work of imagination. While the author's experience with and research of Parkinson's disease have colored these pages, the medical scenarios, symptoms, treatments, and situations exist to serve the story, not to advise.

The author is not a physician or healthcare provider. This book offers no medical guidance and does not promise a cure.

No two people experience Parkinson's the same way. If you're seeking understanding of the disease for yourself or a loved one, please turn to medical professionals who can address your unique circumstances.

Fiction can illuminate truths, but it shouldn't be the basis of healthcare decisions. Read this as a story, because that's what it is.

CHAPTER 1

Saturday, April 25

The moment went on for longer than it should have, for a man standing at a counter with nothing left to do there. Long enough that I noticed it, and then noticed that I had noticed it, and then looked back at my coffee before he turned around.

He picked up the folded paper and slid it into his pocket. "I'll get the tape today. On my way back from the hardware store." He went to the coffeemaker and filled his mug. "And we're out of your bottled water."

"I can get it."

"I'll get it." He came to the table and sat across from me. He read something on his phone. Set it face down. "Father Brennan is leaving," he said.

I looked up.

He turned his mug, making a small circle, clockwise and back. "The Bishop is sending someone from overseas. A missionary. Thirty-two years old." He said it the way he said things he had already formed an opinion about.

“When did you hear this?”

“Kowalski told me at the hardware store on Thursday. He's on the parish council.” Paul's jaw shifted slightly. “Thirty-two years old. Doesn't know anyone. Doesn't know the neighborhood, the families, what the place has been through.” He looked at his coffee. “Father Brennan baptized half the children on this block.”

“He baptized the Kowalski grandchildren,” I said.

“Three of them.” He turned the mug again. “They're sending a stranger to do a job that belongs to someone who knows the people.”

I watched him look at his coffee. He was not a man who went to mass with any regularity. He had not been to church since my diagnosis. The offense he was taking on behalf of a parish he rarely attended was entirely genuine, which was the thing about Paul — his convictions arrived fully formed and didn't require personal involvement to feel absolute.

“Maybe he'll surprise everyone,” I said, wondering if that meant we’d start attending church again...if we could go back to the life we once knew.

Paul looked at his coffee. “Maybe.” His tone said: unlikely.

I took a sip of my coffee. I wasn’t sure we'd find our way back.

CHAPTER 2

Sunday, April 26

"The second shelf," Paul said, "is the problem."

He was standing at the open medicine cabinet with his back to me, his reading glasses on, a legal pad in his left hand. He had been standing there long enough for the coffeemaker to finish cycling. The coffee was ready, but he hadn't moved.

"The organization is gone," he said. "We're treating it like a junk drawer."

I sat at the kitchen table with my hands around my mug and said nothing. There was a system coming. There was always a system.

"Daily medications, front left. As-needed, front right. Supplements behind. Backup supply in the hall closet, labeled." He made a note. "I'll need to pick up label maker tape."

"We have label maker tape."

"It's dried out." Another note. "Also, the childproof caps. Those need to go."

"Paul."

"They're not a safety issue for us. They're an obstacle." He turned and looked at me over his glasses. "How many times have you had trouble with them in the morning?"

I looked at my coffee.

"That's what I thought."

He turned back to the cabinet. The legal pad had three columns. I could see them from where I sat, but not well enough to read them. I didn't need to.

Outside, sunlight made everything look fresh. The maple in the front yard had leafed out after slowly waking up from its long nap. I watched the tree changing for the past two weeks. This morning the leaves were very green.

Paul made another note. I understood this as love. The notes, the systems, the legal pad on a Sunday morning — this was how he said: I am paying attention. I am solving for you. I had learned to read it as clearly as his handwriting, which was an engineer's handwriting, precise and small.

"The morning medications," he said. "You've been taking them with heavy cream in your coffee. The instructions say avoid taking with protein."

"I know what the instructions say."

He wrote something. "I'll put your pills on the kitchen table the night before. With water. So, coffee isn't the nearest thing."

The coffee in my hands was warm. I took a sip.

"Joy."

"I heard you."

He wrote something else. I watched the back of his neck, the set of his shoulders that meant he was concentrating on a problem he intended to resolve before he put the legal pad down.

His hair had gone mostly gray in the last few years. I had watched it happen season by season and said nothing, because he hadn't mentioned it and we had an unspoken agreement about certain categories of change.

"The pill cutter," Paul said. "Where is it?"

"Second drawer."

He said, "It was in the third drawer."

"I moved it."

"When did you move it?"

"Last month."

He wrote something on the legal pad. Updating his catalog of the house. He did this automatically, the way other people breathed — running an inventory of everything we owned and where it lived. When we first got married, I found this quality useful, then maddening. I was now somewhere between both.

"Okay." He closed the cabinet. Took off the reading glasses, folded them, and slid them into his shirt pocket. He tore the top sheet off, folded it twice, and set it on the counter.

Then he stood there. His hand rested on the counter beside the folded paper. Not moving. He was looking at the cabinet door, or past it — at something I couldn't see from where I sat. His fingers were still. His shoulders had dropped from their working position to something lower and less resolved, the drop that happened when a problem had been organized but not yet closed. He picked up the paper and walked into his office.

Site assessment complete.

CHAPTER 3

Tuesday, May 5

Something is wrong with the water. Every morning at the bathroom sink, a chemical tang coated my sinuses. Sharp and metallic, like something industrial had leached into the pipes.

"It's the chlorine," Paul said when I'd mentioned it. He'd been studying a site plan, not bothering to look up. "Seasonal variations in treatment levels."

"It smells like a chemistry lab exploded."

"That's dramatic."

"Is it? Smell the water."

He looked up and met my eyes. "I did. It smells fine."

Of course it did. Paul's sense of smell had gotten terrible in the last year or so. He couldn't tell the difference between burned toast and fresh coffee. I'd learned not to trust him on questions of scent.

But what if it isn't the water? What if it is my brain?

CHAPTER 4

Friday, May 8

I was walking across the gym parking lot toward the entrance when my right leg stopped working. There had been no warning, just a sudden absence of cooperation, as if my body had stopped telling the truth. The pavement came up fast. Asphalt and copper on my tongue.

Two women rushed over — Lisa and Tammy from the gym. They slowed when they got within five feet.

"Oh my god," Lisa said.

I pushed myself onto my knees. Blood mixed with saliva, metallic and warm.

"Should we call someone?" Tammy asked Lisa, not me. She took a small step back.

"I'm fine," I managed, though blood was dripping from my chin.

Lisa glanced at Tammy. "That was a nasty fall. For no reason."

Tammy's face arranged itself into concern. She raised her voice slightly. “Has this happened before?”

“I tripped,” I said.

“Right. Well, if you're sure you're okay.”

They retreated to their car with their heads bent together. I caught fragments as I stood: *...disoriented... we should... not our place... drugs.*

The women watched me walk to my car but didn't follow.

A scream swelled in my chest. But I bit my tongue when the speech therapist’s reminder came to my mind, so all that came out was a groan. *Speak with intent, but don’t strain your voice.* The therapist had drilled the idea into my head. I'd practiced *intent* for two months—which was the time allowed for therapy by our tier of health insurance. *Don't let your voice disappear.*

CHAPTER 5

Saturday, May 9

From the bathroom, I could hear Paul going through his sequence: mug from the third hook, the creak of the refrigerator door, the drawer opening for a spoon. His chair squeaked when he sat down and got up again.

He never wore slippers, even in January. Going barefoot was a habit from his Pennsylvania childhood that I had stopped arguing with years ago.

Paul's routines were more than habits. They were architecture. The coffee maker needed to be turned on at 5:30. The previous day's newspaper needed to be diagonal to the table's edge, laid down with geometric precision. He arranged the sections in the same order: sports, local news, business.

Once I'd teased him and rearranged the sections. His hand had hovered over the disarranged newspaper, while he fought the urge to reorganize the sections. When he gave in, his shoulders dropped with relief.

Over the years, I'd learned that his routines were holding back stress, like levees against rising water. But this past year, despite his routines, stress was leaking through. He seemed slower, stiffer, and tense.

Last year, I'd moved the measuring spoons to the wrong drawer. He'd spent three minutes opening and closing cabinets. Once I realized what he was looking for, I said, "They're in the third drawer now."

He'd looked at me as if I'd rearranged the laws of physics. "Why would you do that?"

"To see if you'd survive."

He had. Barely.

Last Friday, his office had called. I didn't catch the details — only Paul's voice dropping to the register he used when there was nothing left to negotiate. After the call, he said, "This project is going to kill me."

"Which project is this?"

"Finch Street." He turned off his phone and put it on the counter. "Richards wants me to push it through."

He spent the next twenty minutes reorganizing our spice rack—alphabetically, by height, and then by frequency of use. I watched him calculate. I imagined him thinking, if I arrange the paprika and the parsley in the right way, the project will come together.

He was so intent on organizing the spices that his hand shook. I wanted to reach out and tell him everything would be alright, but I knew he wasn't only worried about work. He was worried about our future, about needing to care for his wife whose brain was betraying them both. I wanted to tell him that I was worried too. I hated what was happening to me.

But if I acknowledged his worry, I'd blurt out my own feelings and make everything worse. So, I watched as he moved the cinnamon.

I could feel the distance between us grow wider than the two feet of kitchen tile separating us. Searching for something to bridge the gap, I blurted out, "I've been thinking about getting a water filter."

He stopped moving the spices and met my eyes. After a few moments, he said, "I'll install filters under both sinks."

But this morning, despite the filter under the bathroom sink, the sharpness still annoyed me. I turned off the faucet and stared at my reflection in the cracked mirror. A bruise had ripened overnight, purple-yellow spreading from my chin to my cheekbone. I tilted my head, examining the damage from another angle. *When I stop finding it funny, that's when I'll be in trouble.*

CHAPTER 6

Saturday, May 9

"Morning, Paul!" I called through the open bathroom door, my voice loud enough to carry to the kitchen, with clear enunciation, like I was presenting to a room.

"Morning, Joy," Paul called back, his voice warm with caffeine and habit. "Did you sleep last night?"

"Like a colicky baby. Woke up every two hours."

"So, it was a good night." He laughed, and I loved the smile in it.

His footsteps approached, soft on the floor. Paul appeared in the bathroom doorway, two mugs in hand.

"Coffee delivery." He set mine on the counter, steam curling up between us.

"You're my favorite person," I said.

I saw his stress when he handed me the coffee. His delivery was nearly as unstable as my own might have been.

"I know." He kissed my nose, avoiding the bruise. A gentle warmth emanated from his lips, mingled with the comforting aroma of coffee and the crisp scent of his daily mint soap.

He said, "Even when you fall and scare the hell out of me."

"It was a tumble."

"It was you hitting the pavement," Paul said. His warm hand found my back. "So yeah. Scared the hell out of me."

I leaned into him. For a moment we stood there, him in his work clothes, me in pajamas.

"Are you okay?" I asked. "Coffee delivery is a bit late."

"Fine," he said. "I've been thinking about work."

I took a sip of coffee and set my white cup on the counter.

"Your bruise is worse," he said.

"Thank you for that astute medical assessment, doctor."

He paused before speaking. "Skip the gym today?"

I shook my head. "No."

He sighed. "Danish?"

"Please."

He grinned, the corners of his eyes crinkling. "You'll need to walk to the kitchen for it."

"Worth the effort?"

He picked up my cup. "They're filled with cheese."

"My favorite kind. How did you know?"

I followed him down the hallway, my hand trailing along the wall. In the kitchen, morning light slanted through the window above the sink, catching the dust in the air. Paul had already set out a plate with two heated Danish pastries, the kind from the bakery on Wolf Blvd. that we treated ourselves to once a week.

I took a bite and closed my eyes. Buttery, flaky, the cheese filling smooth on my tongue. For a moment, everything else fell away—just Paul with his newspaper, morning light through the window, sweet goodness.

"Warm enough?" He asked, not looking up from the sports section. I spotted the corner of his mouth lifting.

"Perfect," I said.

He turned the page. "Took me years to perfect the skill."

I laughed.

His reading glasses slipped down his nose. He'd bought his first pair two years ago when he admitted he couldn't read small print. Lately, he'd forget he was wearing them, sometimes looking for them while they perched on his head. It made me love him more, somehow: these small defeats his body handed him, the way he adapted and forgot he'd adapted.

I took another bite of Danish, watching him read. His lips moved as he worked through an article about the local high school's baseball team. He played baseball in college. He kept his old mitt in a box in the garage, though his throwing arm had given out decades ago. He never talked about it, but sometimes I'd catch him flexing his right shoulder, as if he were testing to see if this time it might be different.

"They're saying Thompson's kid might get scouted," Paul tapped the paper. "The pitcher. Remember him? Came to the house selling wrapping paper for the school fundraiser."

"The tall one with the braces?"

"Kid's got an arm on him." His eyes went distant. The corners of his mouth pulled down and then relaxed again. "Paper says he's throwing ninety miles an hour. At seventeen."

"Is that fast?"

"College scholarship fast." He folded the paper and set it aside, taking a long sip of his coffee. "His dad must be over the moon."

I heard what he didn't say. We would never watch our own kids play sports or spoil grandchildren. We'd tried for years, paid for fertility treatments we couldn't afford, then made an unspoken agreement to stop talking about it.

I finished the last bite of Danish and licked a crumb of sugar from my thumb. Paul watched me do it.

"You've got..." He gestured to his own upper lip.

I wiped my mouth with my napkin. "Better?"

"Better."

Paul unmuted the kitchen TV. "...PharmaGenix voluntary medication recall, fewer than one percent of distributed medications were affected. In other health news, authorities expect periodic water pressure issues this week."

He lowered the volume. "They're always recalling something." He turned back to the sports section.

The news report bothered me, like a mosquito buzzing and pricking.

I picked up my water glass, the one Paul always set up for me, knowing I wouldn't drink it. The liquid appeared clear, but when I raised it to my nose, the idea of taking a sip ran away.

I set it down and picked up my coffee cup. My tongue felt coated. I ran it across my teeth. I thought about the protein shake yesterday. It had left a metallic residue for hours. I'd blamed the whey powder. *Had it been the water?*

"Are you okay?" Paul asked.

I'd been staring at the glass with the coffee cup halfway to my mouth.

"Thinking about going to the gym again," I lied, and took a sip of coffee. "I should get dressed."

I retreated to the bedroom. By the time I'd wrestled into my sports bra and tied my shoes—loops that used to be automatic—twenty minutes had passed. My right hand trembled from the morning's demands: fine, rapid, irritating

Dr. Patel's diagnosis had landed like a closed door: early-onset Parkinson's disease. Polite, final, and not mine to argue with.

I opened the bottle of pills. *There is more to me than this.* I took out a white pill, levodopa, the first-line medication. Our insurance wouldn't pay for the newer drugs.

Dr. Patel had once mentioned them. "The newer dopamine agonists might cause fewer movement problems at the beginning, but they bring their own issues."

I swallowed the pill with water from the bottle on my nightstand, water I'd bought at the store two days ago, not trusting what came from our faucets, despite the new filters.

I touched the bruise on my forehead and winced.

It hurts. Good. Pain means I'm alive.

Paul appeared in the doorway, his coffee cup in hand. "Are you sure about the gym?"

"I'm sure."

"Joy..."

"If I stop going, I won't want to start again."

His jaw worked for a moment.

"You don't want me to get fat, do you?"

"Okay. But if you fall again..."

"I won't."

"But if you do," he said, "you call me."

"Deal."

He left, and I finished getting ready. When I returned to the kitchen, Paul had put my gym bag on the counter. The water bottle was full, and he had put a protein bar in the side pocket.

"You packed my bag?" I asked.

"You were taking forever." But his smile was soft. "Besides, you always forget something."

"I forget things—strategically. It's called delegation."

"It's called I found your water bottle in the fridge next to the milk."

"I was pre-chilling it."

"For three days?"

Yep. He got me.

"Well, thank you."

"Anytime." His finger traced down a column about an industrial site development. He read the paragraph three times. I watched his eyes track the same lines.

"Huh," he said.

His shoulders were rigid and rounded.

"Someone local won the lottery," Paul said. "Guy works at the hardware store on Highland. Worked, I guess. Past tense, now."

He paused, frowning. "Says he moved out of state two weeks after winning." He snorted. "Smart man. Getting out while he could."

The last part came out quieter, as if he hadn't meant to say it aloud.

My eyes kept drifting to the kitchen sink. I went over and turned on the faucet to rinse my coffee cup.

That sharp scent again.

Paul stood, his chair scraping against the tile. "I've got the site..." He paused, his forehead creasing. "Site..."

"Assessments," I said.

"Yeah." He carried his mug to the sink. When he reached past me to rinse it, his hand trembled.

I said, "Are you anxious about something?"

Water splashed onto his cuff. "Nothing I can't handle. The Finch soil samples showed higher levels than expected."

He turned off the water.

"Levels higher? Of what?" I asked.

His fingers drummed against the counter. He'd started doing that about six months ago. Mostly when he was stressed. "Heavy metals. Some chemical compounds we're still identifying."

"Any chance it's in the water?"

Paul understood I had become hyperalert to the water. I couldn't help it. Anyone who smelled what I did would share my worry.

"Nothing to do with our water supply."

Last week you said the Wilcox aquifer is under the entire area.

I didn't say what I had been thinking.

Paul put his hands in his pockets, taking a casual stance. "Peter says his wife is expecting. Second child. He'll angle for my promotion."

"Everyone understands you've earned it," I said.

"Yeah. Yeah, I have." But his voice carried no conviction, and he was staring at the drain like it might have answers. His eyes met mine for a second, and I caught something. Not worry, more like the fear you see in someone who understands what's coming and can't stop it. It was gone a moment later, shuttered behind his usual expression.

What is going on with him?

"I'll be back in about an hour," I said, grabbing my keys.

"Be careful out there," Paul said.

"Always am."

"That's not true."

I smiled back and headed for the door.

Outside, the scent of cut grass from yesterday's mowing mixed with diesel, probably from the garbage truck. I couldn't see the truck, but it usually showed up around the time I left for the gym.

The car started on the second try. I pulled out of the driveway and drove past Mrs. Henderson's place. A van sat in her driveway.

I kept driving, but in the rearview mirror, I spotted Mrs. Henderson standing in the road, her hand raised, waving at me. Her image disappeared, as though the flash had been a mirage formed by the early morning light. Or it was a trick my brain was playing.

CHAPTER 7

Saturday, May 9

Someone erased me.

I stood in the parking lot, staring at the spot where my face had hit the pavement yesterday. The asphalt was clean, probably power-washed, leaving no evidence of my fall.

I pulled the door open and walked inside.

The smell hit me—sharp enough to punch through whatever Parkinson's had scrambled...a sickening sweet floral scent mixed with bleach.

Toxic.

"Good to see you." Marcus stood behind the front desk where he'd been stationed since this place opened. He had lean muscles and old tattoos softening at the edges. He was the kind of reliable presence that made me feel safe.

He glanced at the bruise I hadn't bothered to cover. "Heard about yesterday."

"I'm clumsy."

My gym bag felt heavier. I shifted it to my left shoulder. The strap dug into my collarbone.

"Right." He paused, and I could see him choosing words. "Listen, Joy, I need to—"

I swiped my card before he could finish. The beep cut through whatever he had queued up. I walked toward the locker room. *Whatever Marcus wants to say can wait.*

The women's locker room was empty except for one person at the far end who left without looking up. I shoved my bag into locker 40. The metal door echoed the force I used to shut it.

My reflection stared back at me from the mirror across the room. The lighting added another decade to my fifty-three years, or maybe that was Parkinson's marking me. I ran my hands through my hair, trying to look less like I'd lost a fight with a parking lot. The woman in the mirror didn't cooperate. She never did anymore.

At least I showed up, I thought. *That's what they tell you to do. Show up. Keep moving. Stay positive...Bullshit advice from people whose bodies still work.*

I stepped out of the locker room and onto the weight floor. Metal clanged in steady bursts. Someone nearby huffed through a hard set, and a woman's shoes squeaked across the rubber mats. It was the gym's familiar symphony — a chorus of effort, every sound shaped by people chasing a stronger version of themselves.

A rowing machine nearby clicked and wheezed with every pull. Two women moved in perfect rhythm on the ellipticals, their strides rising and falling together. Across the room, someone powered through leg presses, metal plates slamming hard enough to echo. Overhead, the air conditioning rattled and blew a thin stream of cool air that faded before it ever reached the corners.

I stepped up to the dumbbell rack and wrapped my hand around a ten-pound weight. The cold metal settled into my palm, heavier than I had expected. My arm protested instantly. I exhaled, set it back in place, and reached for an eight instead.

Progress in reverse. The story of my life. Last month I'd been using ten-pound weights. At this rate, by Christmas I'll be training with pool noodles. By spring, feathers. By next summer, I'll just think about lifting weights and call it a day.

A woman stepped off the elliptical near the water fountain. As she reached for her bottle, I noticed the tremor — a rhythm different from mine, but familiar enough that I caught my breath.

Part of me wanted to walk over, to say something that might bridge the distance between us. Another part wanted to turn and disappear into the noise of the room. Instead, I fixed my eyes on the eight-pound dumbbell in my hand and pretended it required all my attention.

A woman's voice said, "You need to breathe."

I turned around. The woman from the elliptical stood behind me. She had rosy cheeks and fine lines radiating from her eyes. A neat ponytail hung to her shoulders. She wore workout clothes that matched in a way mine never did.

"I'm breathing," I said. My words came out more defensively than I'd intended.

"Not enough." She smiled, but it didn't reach her eyes.

She said, "I'm Rebecca."

"Joy."

I set the dumbbell down. We shook hands. I pretended not to notice her slow movement, the way you pretend not to notice a lot of things when your body is betraying you in public.

"Ouch. That must've hurt." She gestured to my forehead.

I touched the bruise. "Parking lot won."

"How long have you had it? The Parkinson's."

"Diagnosed four years ago. Though I think it started earlier. Like five, six years ago." I flexed my right hand, watching the tremor dissipate with the movement.

"One year for me," she said. "Official diagnosis, anyway. But I've been noticing things for three years or so. About the time the water system got fixed."

"The water does smell off," I said.

Her expression shifted. "Lots of things smell off with Parkinson's."

"You smell it too? The water?"

"No. But my nose doesn't work right." She picked up a resistance band someone had tossed onto the rack and stretched it between her hands. The rubber made a soft sound. Her phone started playing the theme song from the Rocky Horror Picture Show.

I laughed. "Time Warp?"

She muted it. "Husband message song."

"Let me guess. His name is—"

"Rocky," we said together.

She smiled. "It's his nickname. Steve."

I laughed. "I like your choice of song."

She said, "I was shocked when I found out I had Parkinson's."

"Me too."

"Thought I was tired, or stressed, or getting old." She paused. "Isn't that what we all do? Make excuses until we can't anymore?"

"What made you stop making excuses?"

Rebecca said, "I couldn't tie my shoes. Sounds stupid, right? I'm a pharmacist. I dispense medications—some cost more than my car. I counsel people on life-threatening conditions. But a shoelace defeated me. I sat on my bathroom floor, crying. My cat walked by and looked at me like I was the saddest thing she'd ever seen."

"Oh, I can relate."

"Thing is, I know the symptoms. But I convinced myself it was something else...right up until those shoelaces."

I nodded. "I used to help my husband with his dress-shirt tie. He called the task a pious act of patience."

Rebecca smiled. "Are you still working?"

"No. Quit three years ago."

Around us, bodies lunged and lifted in steady motion. Sneakers slapped against the rubber floor, and the air carried that sweet-musky scent of effort. I used to move like that — chasing the burn, testing my strength. Now I felt like someone set apart from it all, the person others might glance at with relief, thinking, Thank God that's not me.

Rebecca's gaze shifted to something behind me, and her eyes widened slightly. "Well, I should head home. Nice meeting you."

Before I could respond, a voice came from behind my shoulder.

CHAPTER 8

Saturday, May 9

"Joy, can I talk to you for a minute?"

I turned around to find Marcus standing there, his expression neutral.

"In my office." His voice was too controlled, too careful.

Rebecca walked toward the locker room.

I followed Marcus past the weight machines, past the cardboard cutout fitness model with her impossible abs and gleaming smile, through the door marked Staff Only.

The office smelled of old coffee and printer toner. Metal cabinets were pushed against a wall; with their drawers half-open as if they'd given up on closing. The desk was buried in paperwork and protein bar wrappers.

"I don't want to do this." Marcus picked up a pen and put it down. "Corporate office sent someone last week. Auditing incident reports. Liability prevention." He shook his head. "There was a report filed about your fall yesterday morning. Last night, they flagged it."

"I fell in the parking lot. Outside."

"On gym property." His voice was tight. "Look, I've known you for three years. You've never caused problems. But corporate says the new public health policy states that anyone with an observable impairment needs medical clearance."

"Clearance?"

"That's what corporate says," he added quickly, as if he didn't believe it either.

My fingers found the edge of his desk. The laminate was sticky with something I didn't want to identify. Heat traveled up my arm into my shoulder.

Observable impairment—more like a socially challenging presence.

It was this establishment's polite way of saying I was broken. That I was a liability and made people nervous by exercising in the same space.

"I need documentation from your doctor," Marcus said. "A note saying you're safe to use the facilities unsupervised."

"And if I can't get it?"

"You lose your membership."

"How long do I have?"

"One week."

"I'll get the note."

"Thank you. I am sorry about this."

"You're sorry."

"I am. This isn't personal—"

"It is personal, Marcus. You're telling me other people are uncomfortable having me in the gym."

"That's not—"

"Isn't it?" My hands were shaking harder now. Not from Parkinson's, from anger. "I fell in your parking lot. Not in your gym. Not using your equipment."

Marcus looked lost.

"I'm not dangerous. I have Parkinson's. There's a difference."

"I know there is."

"Do you? Because from where I'm standing, it looks like you're wanting to kick out a person who moves differently."

I stood up. "I'll get your note. But this is not right."

My mother had taught high school English for thirty years. She could quote Dickinson from memory and recite entire acts of Shakespeare while cooking Sunday dinner. Words were her currency, her power, her identity. She taught me to use my words to fight for everything, even when the battle felt small, even if I felt small.

I walked to the door. Turned back. "Everyone is sorry," I said. "Sorry doesn't change anything." I left before he could respond.

Sorry, Mom. It takes energy to find the right words.

The walk back to the weight floor felt longer than it should have. *My legs feel heavier. Everything is heavier.*

I picked up a five-pound dumbbell. Five bicep curls before my arm gave out. I set it down, rested for a minute, and picked it back up. Five more. Halfway through triceps, I switched from five pounds to fours

A woman across the weight floor was watching me. She stared at me, the way people look at car accidents, with horrified fascination and grateful distance. I met her eyes. She looked away. I finished my set but added three more reps to prove I could.

In the locker room, I showered and changed into my street clothes. As I dressed, I imagined that somewhere, people were living normal lives, making plans, and taking their bodies for granted. In my imagined world, no one needed to think about medical clearance forms or observable impairments or whether they'd still be able to button their own shirts next year.

I stuffed my workout clothes into my bag. I'd forgotten to pack deodorant. I'd also forgotten to pack shampoo, a hairbrush, and apparently, dignity. But I had my water bottle, thanks to Paul. *One out of four. Passing grade in some schools.* I walked out past the front desk with my tangled, wet hair. Marcus looked up but didn't say anything. What was there to say?

CHAPTER 9

Thursday, May 14

My mother once said, “Dying is easy. It's getting there that's hard.” She'd been talking about cancer, the way it ate through her body over eighteen months. “Quick deaths are mercies. The slow ones are torture.”

Parkinson's wouldn't kill me—not directly. But it would take everything it could while I was alert enough to watch. If I lived long enough, I’d eventually lose the ability to walk, speak, or swallow. If dementia came first, I wouldn't even have the satisfaction of knowing what I'd lost.

My mother would have said, “Knowing is both better and worse.” She would’ve appreciated the irony. She was big on irony, less so on practical advice. Her suggestions—positive thinking, vegetables—hadn't saved her.

After she died, I sat beside her grave and spoke into the quiet. “Your worldview promised control.” I told her, “But your illness ignored it.” I felt heavier once the words were out. “I don’t have promises of control. All I have is a prophesied prognosis. How am I supposed to live inside this?”

Thursday morning, I was in Dr. Patel's waiting room. It smelled of antiseptic with hints of lavender air freshener that couldn't quite mask the staleness underneath.

An older man sat near the window. His hands refused to rest on his knees. Two fingers made a soft whisper of movement, flesh rubbing against cotton. His face hung slack, the muscles beneath the skin gone still, as if someone had cut the wires.

A woman entered. She was my age, or younger. It was hard to tell. Her hair was pulled up and fastened with a hair clip, in a way that said survival outranked grooming. She approached the receptionist's desk, with her canvas bag slipping off her shoulder.

“I have an appointment about my hand.” Her voice held steady, but the last word pulled tight.

The receptionist kept typing.

The woman said, “It shakes. My husband says it's carpal tunnel. But I'm a professional artist, and...”

The receptionist's fingers stopped typing.

At my first appointment with Dr. Patel, I’d thought the doctor would say it was nothing or stress or menopause related...something that could be fixed with a pill and maybe some physical therapy. I'd been wrong.

The receptionist said, “Have you been here before?”

"No."

The receptionist handed the woman a clipboard. "Have a seat and fill out these forms."

The woman took the clipboard and sat in a chair near a fake plant. The plant looked healthier than most of the people in the waiting room, which said something about the advantages of being plastic.

"Joy Anderson?" I looked over and saw the nurse who had called my name.

The nurse's scrubs were printed with cartoon cats wearing stethoscopes. *No one in this office is a child. Maybe she thinks it will make medical visits feel less medical. Or maybe she lost a bet.*

"Dr. Patel is ready for you."

The woman with the clipboard stopped writing. Her eyes tracked my movements as I stood.

I wish I could tell her—the bruise is facial decoration.

I followed the nurse down the hallway. Fluorescent lights hummed at the edge of hearing—the kind of sound you don't notice until you do. Like my heartbeat when I'm trying to sleep, or my fingers rolling invisible cigarettes.

Anatomical diagrams decorated the walls. Cross-sections of the brain in cheerful pinks and blues. Alongside the diagrams hung motivational posters framed in black and bolted to the wall with anti-theft hardware, as if someone might steal inspirational quotes. *Your only limit is you!* one proclaimed on a picture of a runner crossing a finish line.

My limit is neurons. Chemistry. The death of dopamine-producing cells. But positive thinking? Sure, it might help me win a marathon...if I ever decide to start running.

The nurse led me into room three. "Dr. Patel will be with you in a moment."

I sat on the examination table. The paper sheet crinkled beneath me. The room was painted a shade of beige that might have been called warm sand but looked more like resignation. A poster hung on the wall, positioned for patient contemplation. It showed a mountain climber mid-ascent, his face turned toward an impossibly blue sky, one hand reaching for the next hold. The caption read: *Progress, not perfection.* The climber's muscles were taut, his expression determined, his body obeying every command his brain issued.

During my first visit here, I'd stared at the poster while Dr. Patel explained, "Parkinson's is progressive...there is no cure, only management...dopamine...degeneration...decline."

As the diagnosis landed, I tried to find something hopeful in the idea of climbing a mountain. Now I saw the cruelty of the idea.

On the counter sat a model brain with separated hemispheres, its parts labeled with tiny stickers: red cerebellum, yellow hippocampus, black substantia nigra.

Five minutes passed...then ten. Dr. Patel was never late. In all my appointments, she'd been punctual to the point of predictability. Three minutes early, sometimes. Never late. I stood and crossed to the door, then stopped. *What am I doing?* I was already pressing my ear to the hollow-core surface.

Voices filtered through, muffled but understandable. I heard a woman's voice, younger than Dr. Patel's. "They're going to notice. You're seeing twice as many patients."

I held my breath.

"What about the forms?"

Dr. Patel said, "I'll handle it."

Footsteps retreated with soft squeaks on linoleum.

I sat back down. My heart was pounding hard enough to feel it in my throat. *Twice as many patients. What does that mean?*

The door opened. My neurologist stepped inside. Dr. Patel was in her mid-sixties. She had dark hair pulled into a neat bun and bangs that framed her face. Her white coat was crisp, her name tag catching both light and attention. She held a tablet in her left hand. Her other hand's fingers rolled against each other.

"Mrs. Anderson. Good to see you. How have you been managing?"

"Fine." The word came out automatic, reflexive. Then I reconsidered. "Not great, actually."

She looked up. Her gaze went to the bruise on my face. "What happened?"

"I fell. In the gym parking lot."

Dr. Patel set the tablet down and pulled up a rolling stool. She saw me looking at her hand and tucked it under the other.

"Have you noticed any freezing of gait? It's common with Parkinson's."

I shook my head. "Sometimes my leg doesn't want to do what I tell it to do. It lags. But I wouldn't say I freeze."

"The neural pathways controlling movement become unreliable."

She reached for the tablet again.

The conversation I'd overheard kept repeating in my head. *Twice as many patients.*

"We may need to adjust your dosage. Falls are a concern. Any other new symptoms?"

"Dr. Patel, have you noticed an increase in Parkinson's patients?"

She set her tablet down. When she met my eyes, her expression had shifted.

"Yes," she said. "I've seen an increase. Parkinson's is increasing everywhere."

Her directness surprised me.

"Now, what brought you in today? Besides the fall."

"The gym needs medical clearance. A note saying I'm safe to use the facilities."

"After you fell on their property."

"Yes."

Dr. Patel was quiet for a moment. When she spoke, her voice was measured. "I can't give you full clearance, Joy. Not because I don't believe in you. I do. But the liability framework puts both of us at risk."

The explanation didn't seem like a refusal. But in effect, it was.

"So that's it?"

She reached for her prescription pad. "I'm going to give you something that protects both of us. Limited clearance. No equipment that requires balance unless supervised. It should be enough to keep your membership, but not enough to make either of us liable if something happens."

She began writing.

I said, "I need the gym, Dr. Patel. It's the only place where I still feel like myself."

She looked up from the pad. “I understand that.”

“You have it too, don't you?”

She stopped writing. For a moment, she didn't move.

“February. The tremor started in February.”

“So, you're—”

“Living it. Yes.” She met my eyes. “When I tell you that exercise matters, or talk about managing symptoms and preserving function, I'm not just your doctor. I'm someone who understands what you're going through.”

Two women with the same disease: different stages, same enemy.

She tore off the note and handed it to me.

“So, when you tell me the levodopa helps?”

Dr. Patel glanced up from the chart. “How’s the timing going — still three times a day? And the extended at night?”

“When I remember.”

“Memory problems?”

“No. Resistance.” I gave a small shrug. “Every pill feels like an admission that I’m sick. Some days I’m not ready to say it out loud, even to myself. So, the dose slips later than it should, sometimes up to an hour late.” I flicked my fingers, hoping to stop the tremor.

I said, “Eventually the shaking convinces me to cooperate. And sometimes it demands I take a pill a bit early.”

Her expression softened. “I understand.” She added, “You're the first patient who's admitted that.”

I said, “The levodopa helped at first. My tremor decreased. I could button shirts again. But lately, I've noticed it's wearing off faster.”

“That is a common problem. But there are ways to handle wearing off. At least for a while. We could increase your levodopa.”

“Doesn't that increase my risk of side effects? Like dyskinesia?”

“Yes. But there are options available that might help.”

“If you weren't my doctor,” I said, “if you were speaking only as someone who had Parkinson's, what would you tell me?”

She paused. “I'd tell you that the typical medical approach to Parkinson's is, in many cases, inadequate.”

I folded the note for the gym and put it in my pocket. “What do you mean?”

She glanced at the door, then back at me.

Dr. Patel took a business card out of her coat pocket. She held it for a moment, turned it over and wrote something on the back before handing it to me.

“How do you manage your symptoms?” I asked.

“Levodopa can be effective for some people. It can help when symptoms interfere with daily activities. But it will not slow the progression.”

“Do you take it?”

She let out a slow breath. “No. I don't.”

“Why not?”

“My symptoms are manageable for now. When they're not, levodopa will be there. It's a timing decision.”

She added, “People with Parkinson's still produce some dopamine in the earlier stages. I'm choosing an alternative approach for now. Focusing on other strategies to manage symptoms and preserve function.”

“What kind of strategies?”

She met my eyes. “Treatment decisions are individualized.”

“Maybe I shouldn't be taking levodopa,” I said.

“Only you can know if levodopa is effective for you. But the standard of care dictates that the proper treatment of Parkinson's usually includes levodopa.”

“What if I didn't want to use levodopa anymore?”

“If you ever wanted to stop levodopa, you'd need medical supervision. Tapering down is essential. Stopping suddenly can cause irreversible damage, even death.”

“What if I wanted to talk to someone about treatment options? Outside of this office?”

She stood and walked to the door. Opened it.

“I'll see you in six months. Unless things change.” She turned back, her face composed and professional. “If they do, call.”

She said, “If the gym isn't working out, there are other options. Places that understand movement disorders. Exercise is the only proven medicine that may slow the progression of Parkinson's.”

Is exercise medicine?

I looked down at the card. A phone number was written across the back, and below it, three words in small, careful handwriting: "Trust your instincts." And scribbled, like an afterthought, "Rock Steady Boxing."

She opened the door wider and left.

CHAPTER 10

Wednesday, June 3

Paul had made dinner. This was not unusual. Paul cooked when he worked from home — a habit so established it had become expected. Tonight, it was chicken. I was tired of chicken. This time, it was something with lemon. It smelled right, but I wasn't hungry, which had nothing to do with the chicken.

I sat at the table and Paul set the plate in front of me.

"You didn't eat lunch," he said.

"I had something."

"What did you have?"

It wasn't a question...the register of a man taking inventory.

"Crackers," I said.

He cut his chicken.

"And coffee."

"That's not lunch."

“It was lunch-like.” I watched for the almost-smile. It came — the corner of his mouth, briefly — and then it didn't. He looked back at his plate.

“Dr. Patel’s card is still on the counter,” he said.

I took a bite of chicken. It was good.

“I know,” I said.

“Two weeks.”

“I know how long it's been, Paul.”

He set his fork down. “I'm not criticizing.”

“You're counting.”

“I'm concerned.”

The sprinkler outside ran its cycle. The evening hadn't decided to cool down yet. Paul picked his fork back up and simply held it.

“She wrote a phone number on it,” I said. “That means something.”

“It means you should call.”

“It means I'll call when I'm ready.”

“You've been ready for two weeks.”

I looked at him. “That's not fair,” I said.

He said, “I'm not trying to be—be...to fight you.”

He stopped again.

Then he said, “You've been taking your medication late.”

“Some mornings,” I said.

“Most mornings.” He said it the way he reported findings. “An hour late. Sometimes more. I've noticed how you move before it kicks-in. The pills help.”

“You've been watching me.”

“I live with you.”

"You've been tracking me."

"I've been worried about you." The words came out with more weight than he intended. He heard it and set his fork down. "The timing matters, Joy. You know that. Wearing off, waiting too long, it could make you feel...feel. You should take it on time."

"I know what wearing off feels like. I'm the one wearing off."

"Then why?"

"Because every pill is an admission." I heard my voice sharpen. "Every pill is me saying out loud, again, that this is real. Some mornings I'm not ready to say it. You don't get to decide when I'm ready."

He was quiet for a moment. "You're right," he said. "I don't."

But he didn't stop the lecture. "You've been sleeping late," he said. "The last month. It takes you longer to get going in the morning. I've been starting work late."

I looked at him. "What?"

"Forty minutes. Sometimes an hour."

"Paul. I didn't ask you to do that."

"I know you didn't."

"Why didn't you say something?"

"Because you would have told me not to." He said it simply. He was right, which made it worse. "Because you would have set your alarm for six and gotten up and pushed through, and that would have been harder on you than the extra time."

"You don't get to make that decision."

"Someone had to."

"I am someone." The words came out before I knew how much I meant them. I heard them in the room between us. Paul heard them.

"You're managing me," I said. "The card, the medication, the mornings — you're running your system on me, but I am not a project."

"You know how I am. I count things," he said. "I track things. That's what I do." It was a plain statement of fact about himself. "I don't know what else to do when I'm—" He stopped and looked at the table. "When I watch you and I can't—"

He didn't finish.

He looked at his plate. At the chicken he hadn't eaten.

"Fix it," he said.

The word sat between us.

I looked at my hands on the table. Not checking them. Just looking at them, the way you looked at something that had always been there.

"I know you can't fix it," I said.

"I know you know." He looked up. "That doesn't make it easier to stop trying."

I didn't say anything. The fight had gone somewhere neither of us had planned.

Paul stood. He picked up our plates and carried them to the sink without comment.

"I'll do the dishes," I said.

"I've got them."

"Let me do the dishes."

He turned. A long look — that was using the last ten minutes as its surface. "Okay."

He left the kitchen. His footsteps went down the hall and the office door opened and did not close. He usually left the door open so he could hear the house.

I stood at the sink. The water was warm. I ran it over the plates and put them into the dishwasher. I dried my hands on the towel he had used. I stood at the counter and looked at Dr. Patel's card.

Then, I went into the living room, to the piano. I stood with my hand on the lid, not opening it, not stepping away.

CHAPTER 11

Friday, June 5

I picked up the card a dozen times, turned it over, read the three words on the back—Trust your instincts—then set it down again. The corners were starting to soften, the edges no longer sharp.

I knew Paul was tracking what I was doing. I didn't care. I tucked the card between a stack of unread mail and the shallow bowl of lemons. The envelopes leaned together, unopened. The lemons had gone soft at the ends, their skins dulled. I noticed all of this without doing anything about it.

Paul was loading the dishwasher. This was notable because Paul rarely loaded the dishwasher. When he washed the dishes, he usually did them by hand.

When he unloaded the dishwasher, he'd do it with careful precision, stacking plates by size, aligning cups so their handles faced the same direction. Loading, however, had always been my domain.

A dish rattled against its neighbors. He was putting plates in the wrong slots. Bowls where cups should go. Mugs tilted at angles that made no sense. Everything was incorrect, as if he were staging a domestic rebellion.

"That's not how you load a dishwasher," I said.

"I've been loading dishwashers for twenty years," he replied.

"Incorrectly."

He put another bowl into a space meant for plates.

"Are you dishwasher-shaming me?" he asked.

"I'm dishwasher-educating you."

"Is that what you're calling it?" He flicked water at me from the plate he was rinsing.

I gasped. "Did you just—"

He did it again, grinning like a man who had rediscovered a reliable source of amusement.

I grabbed the spray nozzle. "Paul. Don't."

"Don't what?" He backed away, hands raised in surrender.

"Don't make me use this."

"You wouldn't."

"I would."

I did. I sprayed him right in the chest and face, soaking his shirt through.

We stared at each other. I was surprised by my own follow-through. Then we both started laughing. My laugh came from deep in my chest.

"Surrender?" I said, still laughing.

"Truce."

We stood there, Paul dripping water on the kitchen floor. He pulled me against his wet shirt. I felt his breath coming fast. Not from the brief excitement of a water fight.

"When did we stop doing this?" he whispered against my hair.

"Fighting?"

"Being stupid together. Having fun. Not thinking about..." He didn't finish.

I pulled back to look at him. Water dripped from his hair onto his nose. His eyes were wet.

"We can still be stupid," I said.

"Do you still want to?" He kissed my forehead. Held me for another moment. Neither of us mentioned the way I'd nearly lost my balance when he'd pulled me close.

Paul stepped back and surveyed the dishwasher, hands on his hips, squinting slightly, the way he did when studying blueprints without his glasses.

"I think my system has merit," he said.

"You don't have a system," I replied. "You have chaos with confidence."

"Explain to me why bowls cannot go here."

"Because they don't belong there."

"That's not a reason."

"It is the reason," I said. "Some things work because they have always worked."

He laughed and rearranged our plates. They leaned against each other at an angle that made my teeth ache. He had once spent forty minutes explaining load distribution to me using saltshakers and napkins. Apparently, glassware was exempt from the laws of physics.

"There," he said. "Improved."

"You're doing this to provoke me."

"I'm doing this to expand your mind."

"My mind is fine," I said. "It's your understanding of basic mechanics that concerns me."

He reached for another plate. I intercepted it and placed it where it belonged. Our hands bumped together.

"It's remarkable how a man who can design drainage systems can't be trusted with dishes."

"You know," he said, smiling, "we could just let it be wrong. Trust the dishwasher to do its job."

"No," I said. "That would be irresponsible."

He raised an eyebrow. "Dishwasher irresponsibility?"

"Absolutely," I said. "It starts small."

Paul shook his head and stepped aside with a theatrical bow. "Fine. Lead the way."

I rearranged the remaining dishes, narrating my choices with exaggerated seriousness. He listened, nodding solemnly, as if committing the information to memory.

Paul turned to the sink and rinsed his hands longer than necessary, adjusting the faucet until the stream ran exactly the way he wanted. The soap dispenser sat by the basin, its label peeling. As he worked the soap between his fingers, the scent filled the air—lavender edged with something sharper underneath.

"I noticed your levodopa is getting low," he said. "You want me to pick up your prescription?"

He pointed the sprayer at me. The soap still coated his hands.

I stepped back toward the doorway. "It's warm out. I think I'll walk to the pharmacy."

"Oh," he said. "Strategic retreat?"

"Exactly."

I grabbed my keys from the table.

"Perfect escape plan," I said.

"Don't take all day," he said. "I actually have a day off for once." He was rinsing lingering bubbles off his fingers.

"While I'm gone, maybe you can dry off."

"While you're gone," he said, "maybe I'll reload the dishwasher."

He stepped over to me, his hands still dripping. Paul brushed hair from my face. His thumb lingered on my cheek.

"You're beautiful when you're armed and dangerous," he said.

"I attacked you."

"Still beautiful."

"Paul," I said. "You're wet."

"I know," he said. "Are you?"

I pressed my face into his wet shirt. "I am now."

He pushed me gently toward the door. "Get going before it gets hotter. And before I get even."

Despite my damp shirt, the afternoon heat was thick enough to feel. Our street looked exactly the way it always had. Neat lawns rimmed with trimmed hedges, surrounding houses full of people paying for the futures they'd imagined. Wind chimes hung from nearly every porch. Glass. Metal. Driftwood. I had never liked them. The sound felt intrusive, as though the air itself was being interrupted.

Mr. Stevens was washing his car. Again. He held the hose with both hands, directing the spray. Water pooled at the curb, overflowing the gutter and running farther down the street. The rear bumper had dulled to gray, as though it had been scrubbed too many times with the wrong sponge.

When he noticed me, he bent closer to the car and worked the sponge over the same section again, slow and methodical. Four years of being neighborly...then Paul told him about my diagnosis, and suddenly his car warranted full devotion.

I kept walking.

Mrs. Henderson's house came into view: pale yellow, white shutters, and a yard that used to win awards. The roses that lined her walkway were brown now, their stems brittle, leaves curled inward as if in retreat. Petals littered the mulch like the remains of a celebration no one had enjoyed. A garden club trophy sat in her front window. A hose lay coiled beneath the spigot.

Why doesn't she water her roses?

Her wind chimes hung from the maple tree, one strand twisted out of alignment and tangled up with a dried leaf. The chime's pieces clacked together instead of ringing.

I tried to remember the last time I had seen Mrs. Henderson outside. *The farmer's market, maybe.*

I walked the rest of the way to the pharmacy without stopping. Mrs. Henderson's wind chimes followed me part of the way; the sound uneven, arriving in short, hollow knocks that never quite resolved into music. When I reached the corner, the noise dropped away, replaced by traffic and the steady hum of an overworked air conditioner.

The automatic doors slid open as I approached, releasing a rush of refrigerated air. I stepped inside. The pharmacy was busier than usual. I took my place at the end of the line and waited. Two women stood in front of me, angled toward each other.

"Sixty dollars for a thirty-day supply," one of them said. "Last year it was forty. The year before that, thirty."

"At this rate," the other said, "I'll be choosing between medication and groceries."

Her friend nodded. "I'm thinking of switching to mail-order."

When the line moved forward, I stepped up to the counter. For three months, Janet had been the one handing over my prescription. Today she was gone. In her place stood Rebecca from the gym.

"Joy, right?" She said, smiling. "I didn't know you came to this location."

"When did you start here?"

"Last week." She turned back to the computer.

"Janet's gone today?"

"Out sick. What can I get you?"

"Refill for Anderson."

Her fingers moved across the keyboard. "Carbidopa-levodopa?"

"That's it."

"Give me just a minute."

She disappeared into the back, leaving me time to explore the greeting card display: Father's Day cards, birthday cards, anniversary cards, and promises printed in glossy ink that were cheerful and confident. One card caught my eye. Two cartoon figures with pear-like faces were tangled in a garden hose, as water sprayed everywhere. *We Make a Great, but Tangled, Pear.*

Paul would think it was stupid. He would also love it. I took it off the rack. The decision was easy.

When Rebecca returned with the white paper bag, she glanced at the card and smiled. "That's cute."

"We had a water fight this morning," I said. "It seemed appropriate."

"Who won?"

"I did," I said. "He's home drying off."

She laughed and rang up the prescription and the card, then paused, her hand resting on the counter. "There's a support group that meets at the community center on Tuesday mornings. People with Parkinson's and their families."

I nodded.

"Maybe I'll come," I said, not really meaning it.

"No pressure," she said. "Just thought I'd mention it. There are support services available."

"Thanks for letting me know."

Outside, the heat hadn't improved. I walked home the way I had come, with the prescription bag in one hand and Paul's card in the other.

Mrs. Henderson's curtains were still drawn.

Her roses are dead.

I slowed at the end of her driveway and stopped. My mind supplied details I hadn't asked for: Mrs. Henderson on the kitchen floor, the phone just out of reach. The roses were left to die not because they were forgotten, but because no one was left to tend them.

I pushed the thought away as soon as it arrived.

But people don't let award-winning gardens die for no reason. I should check on her. That is what neighbors do.

I kept walking.

When I got home, Paul was in the living room, wearing dry clothes and folding laundry. Each towel was squared before being stacked.

"You're doing it wrong," I said.

He looked up and grinned. "Is this another educational moment?"

"No," I said. "You're doing it right. I just wanted to start another fight."

"How was the walk?"

"Hot," I said. "Long. I got you something."

I sat beside him and handed him the card.

He opened it, read it, and his face brightened. "We do make a great pair."

"Even when we're idiots."

"Especially then."

He set the card aside and pulled me against him. My head found the familiar place on his shoulder. His hand moved slowly against my back. The prescription bag sat unopened on the coffee table.

"I love you," I said.

"I love you too," he said. "Even though you tried to drown me."

"That was self-defense."

He said, "That was assault with a deadly nozzle."

The afternoon light moved across the floor. The laundry remained half-folded.

Across the street, Mrs. Henderson's hose lay unused.

CHAPTER 12

Saturday, June 13

A week later, I stood at Mrs. Henderson's door, my hand still raised from knocking, wondering what had changed to make me insert myself into a situation.

The peephole darkened. The door remained closed.

Well, she's not stuck on the floor.

I could leave. Walk back down the driveway, past the dead roses, to my own house and mind my own business. I almost had — twice — stopping on the sidewalk while the bag of tomatoes swung at my side like a quiet argument I hadn't agreed to yet.

An hour earlier, I'd been at the farmers' market. I spotted Mrs. Henderson. She was lifting Cherokee Purples one by one, turning them under the sun.

When she noticed me approaching, she smiled and said, "Heirloom varieties are—" In mid-sentence, her shaking hands let the tomatoes fall.

They burst against the pavement with a soft, rupturing smack that turned a few heads and made a child laugh before his mother pulled him away. Mrs. Henderson stood over the mess, one hand curved as if it still held a tomato. She didn't rush to apologize or clean up. She only watched the red spread between the cracks in the concrete, studying what remained the same way she'd studied the fruit intact.

Mrs. Henderson looked down at her hands as if they belonged to someone else and walked away without a word.

I'd decided not to get involved.

But good sense vanished before I got home. So, here I was.

Why am I still standing here?

The deadbolt clicked. The door opened a crack.

"Mrs. Henderson? It's Joy. From across the street."

The visible sliver of her face shifted. "Joy? What are you doing here? Come inside."

The chain rattled. The door swung open.

Sarah Henderson looked smaller than I remembered. Her reading glasses hung on a chain around her neck. She wore a cardigan despite the heat. Her arms were crossed tightly over her chest. Behind her, the house was in shadow.

I stepped across the threshold. She closed the door and engaged both locks. I was welcomed by Earl Grey and old books, but underneath was something sweet and stale at the same time, like fruit forgotten in a bowl — familiar in a way I didn't want to examine. Paul had started opening our bedroom window every morning. He said it was for fresh air.

Mrs. Henderson's living room curtains were drawn against the afternoon sun. A dusty laptop sat closed on the coffee table. Newspapers were stacked beside the wall, their edges yellowing.

I thought about the unread mail on our counter — and Dr. Patel's card hidden there.

"Would you like some water?" Her voice was quieter than I had expected. I leaned slightly forward. She moved toward the kitchen without waiting for an answer.

I followed her down the hallway — small, careful steps, arms quiet at her sides, each movement considered before it was made — and stepped over a pair of slippers abandoned on the floor. One had landed upside down. The other had been kicked to the wall, its toe pointing back toward the bedroom, trying to return home on its own.

In the kitchen, she pulled a glass from the dish rack — a deliberate reach, her whole body settling into the task. Her hands shook as she filled the glass from the tap. Water sloshed over the rim, spreading across the laminate countertop in a widening pool. She wrapped both hands around the glass and lifted it to her lips. Water dripped down her chin. She didn't wipe it away.

I thought about Paul handing me my coffee mug this morning, his stress-induced shake sloshing the liquid. He watched as I took it from him. I'd gripped it with both hands just to be safe. There was relief in his eyes when I set it down without spilling.

Mrs. Henderson set the glass down and steadied it with both palms.

"You're not here about my cat, are you?"

The question came out casually, as though she was asking about the weather.

"Your cat?"

"Whiskers. She's been missing for days. I put food out, but she hasn't come home." She gestured toward a dish in the corner by the refrigerator.

The dish was there. The cat's food was black with mold.

If Whiskers comes back, she'll take one look at that and choose to stay dead.

Yesterday, I found a container of leftover pasta in our refrigerator. It had been pushed to the back and was so old that the noodles had turned gray.

Paul said, "It's been there for over a month." He opened it, looked at me, and said, "I think it's sentient now. We should name it."

"Harold," I'd said.

"Harold the Pasta Monster. It has a nice ring to it."

We threw Harold away with full funeral honors. Paul had even hummed a hymn.

Mrs. Henderson was looking in her cupboards. "Here kitty. Whiskers. Joy is here. Come say hi."

"Mrs. Henderson. Whiskers died. We buried her together in your backyard. I helped you dig the hole."

She closed the cupboard door. "Of course. I know that. Sometimes I get confused."

Mrs. Henderson's chair scraped against the linoleum, the sound sharp and prolonged, like fingernails on glass. I pulled out another chair and set the bag of tomatoes on the table between us.

Bills were scattered across the table's surface alongside unopened envelopes. A prescription bottle lay on its side, the label turned away from me. I couldn't read the name, but I could see the orange warning sticker. Beside the bills sat a manila folder, its edges soft with handling. Mrs. Henderson sat down and rested her hand on top of it.

"How have you been, Mrs. Henderson?"

"Fine. Just fine."

Is "fine" her word or mine?

She said, "How have you been?"

"Fine. Some days are better than others."

Her gaze drifted to the window above the sink, then back to me. "My daughter visited last week. Or maybe two weeks ago. She worries."

"That's natural."

"She thinks I'm losing my mind." Mrs. Henderson said it like mentioning she'd bought milk at the store. "She may be right. I'm not sure I'm a reliable judge."

I watched her fingers drum against the table. I knew the rhythm. It was Paul's stress-drumming. It was my own hands, sometimes, when the tremor found somewhere new to go.

"How would you know?" she asked. "If your mind is going, can you trust it to tell you the truth about itself?"

The drumming continued. Rhythmic. Automatic.

"No," I said. "I don't think you can."

Her fingers stopped drumming. "Your husband seems nice. I sometimes see him working in your yard. Taking care of things."

"He is. Very attentive."

This morning had been rough. I'd taken my little white pill, but for twenty minutes I was off, waiting for the levodopa to kick in. Paul tied my shoes without commenting. Then tied them in double knots like I was five years old heading to kindergarten. I'd considered protesting.

Is this what Paul sees when he looks at me? Someone who needs tending?

Last week I had a bad day. The medication wasn't working. Paul started cutting my food at dinner without me asking, then pretended he was doing it for himself, rearranging portions on his own plate. Neither of us said anything.

"That's important." Mrs. Henderson's voice pulled me back. "When you can't trust yourself anymore, you need someone who can be trusted."

We sat with that for a moment.

Then she said, "I stopped going out."

She hadn't announced this. It arrived the same way she'd said that her daughter thought she was losing her mind.

"When did you stop?" I asked.

"I'm not sure. It happened in pieces." She looked at the curtained window. "First, I stopped going in the evenings. Then I stopped driving. Then the market became difficult — all those people moving quickly, all that noise. I could never remember what I came for by the time I got there. Today I went because — I don't know why I went today. Something made me go."

She folded her hands on the table. Her hands trembled.

She looked at me then.

I knew what that look was. I'd catalogued it for four years. The careful face. The face that meant, *I see you are not what you were, and I don't know what to do with that information.*

"I might stop going to the gym," I said. "I'm not exercising as much anyway." I looked at the table between us.

Mrs. Henderson was quiet.

"I used to love working out," I said. "Now I can't be there without being the person everyone watches."

"My roses are dead," she said after a moment. "I let them die."

"They were beautiful."

"I used to win awards. Best in the neighborhood." She looked at my hands. "I guess you can't water my roses either, poor dear."

"Is it hard for you to water the roses?"

"I keep thinking I'll water them." She didn't say it with grief, exactly. With the flatness of someone naming a thing they've already spent their grief on. "Things die, I suppose."

My piano came to mind. Months of walking past it, telling myself I'd play it again when the tremor steadied, when I felt more like myself, when the day was the right kind of day. The piano had no opinion about any of this. It remained patient as furniture. Which was the same as waiting forever.

"My daughter says I should sell the house," Mrs. Henderson continued. "Move into one of those places where people take care of you. Where you don't have to worry about bills or gardens or whether you're remembering things correctly."

Paul had mentioned it once before his trip to Phoenix, a retirement community that specialized in neurological conditions. He'd brought home a brochure, left it on the table beside his cup of coffee, and gone into his office to make a call.

"Is that what you want?" I asked.

"I want to tend things," she said. "That's what I want. I want to still be someone who has roses." She looked up at me. "But you can't have a rose bush in a place like that. You can't even tend yourself — someone else does the tending. And then what are you?"

She stood then, slowly. "It's out there. Back there." She crossed to the window and pulled back the corner of the curtain with two fingers. I could tell she wasn't checking for anything. She was just looking at the backyard where a garden had been. "It doesn't matter if it's gone."

She let the curtain fall.

“The doing is the point,” she said to the curtain, or to herself, or to me. “It's not what I can manage to do while I'm there. Just the going.”

I stood. “Speaking of going, I should go home.”

She walked me to the door — the same small, careful steps, arms quiet at her sides. Unlocked the deadbolt, then the chain. I stepped onto the porch. The sunlight felt startling after the dimness inside.

“Thank you for visiting,” she said. “Most people don't anymore.”

I nodded. Then I walked down the porch steps, past the dead roses, back across the street.

Behind me, I heard her door close — both locks, in order, careful and deliberate. The sound of someone's world closing.

CHAPTER 13

Saturday, June 13

The house was exactly as I had left it. I made coffee and stood at the kitchen window, watching a robin investigate the yard. The creature had no concept of the word *prognosis*. It stopped beside the garden bed and cocked its head, listening to something under the surface. I turned away from the window.

On the counter sat a bottle of water I had bought earlier that morning. I bought it because control had gotten very small lately, and buying water was something I could still do with my own hands, without assistance, without being observed doing it, and some mornings that was enough of a reason to do something...anything.

Paul's footsteps crossed from his office to the kitchen — the slightly slower pattern I had been tracking without meaning to track. He appeared in the doorway, his work shirt half-untucked, a site plan in one hand.

"Coffee still hot?" he asked.

"Just made it."

He poured a cup. "The Finch Street report."

He set the site plan on the table. His finger moved to a section near the bottom, then away. "Richards says my assessment parameters are wrong. That I used the wrong baseline for the structural analysis. If I'd run the numbers the new way, the findings would be different." His jaw tightened. "He wants me to redo it. His way."

"And would the findings be different?"

"Possibly. I don't know. Maybe." He looked at the site plan without looking at it. "That's the problem. I ran it the way I was trained to run it. Richards says my methodology is outdated. He might be right."

"What does he want you to do?"

"Reassess using his parameters. Submit a revised report. Sign my name to conclusions I reached using a method I didn't choose and don't entirely trust." He set his coffee down. "If I do it, the report will probably change. That way the project will move forward. I'll get the promotion. If I don't, Richards finds someone who will. Peter, probably. Peter will use whatever parameters Richards gives him."

I watched him reach for the site plan again, smoothing a corner that did not need smoothing.

"You are going to do it," I said.

"I don't know what else to do. If I push back, I become the person who won't cooperate." His fingers were doing the thing on the table, the drumming. "We need insurance. We need the income. You need me to be employed, not fighting a battle I'm not even sure I can win."

"Paul."

"I know what you are going to say."

"Do you?"

"That I should trust my own judgment. That I've been doing this for twenty years and I know what I know." He sat down across from me. "But what if I don't anymore?"

"Making yourself smaller does not make the problem smaller," I said. "It just makes you smaller."

"Richards has been asking me to adjust things for two years. And now I am here." He took a sip, set the cup down, and sighed. "I don't know when I stopped trusting myself. I don't remember the moment. It happened in pieces."

"Write the honest report," I said. "Your way. Document your methodology, explain your reasoning, put your name on the version you believe is accurate, and let Richards decide what to do with it."

"Even if it means I lose my job?"

"Write the honest report. Whatever happens after that, you will have been the person who told the truth when he could."

Paul sat with this. Outside the kitchen window, the robin had moved on.

"You make it sound simple," he said.

"It's not simple. It costs something." I knew what I was asking. I was asking him to risk his career.

"But the alternative also costs something," I said. "It just charges you later, when you're not expecting it."

"When did you get so certain about things?" he asked.

I thought about Mrs. Henderson's front door this morning. "I'm not certain about anything. I'm just telling you what I think is right."

We sat there. The afternoon had gone the color of weak tea, the low lateral light moving across the table between us.

Then Paul said, "I should make tea. It's late for you to be drinking coffee."

"Tea would be good." I kept drinking my coffee.

He stood and went to the counter and filled the kettle — from the tap, without thinking about it, the way you did when water was simply water and didn't smell. The bottled water was on the counter; along with the reassurance it offered.

There's nothing wrong with the water. I'm the only one who smells it.

He took a mug down, my extra one, the one Paul bought for me, *just in case.* He rinsed his blue one. Set them side by side with the handles facing out. Then he turned back to the kettle and stood watching it, which was something he had always done and always said was pointless. *Watched water* and all of that. He watched it anyway, every time, because some habits had nothing to do with efficiency and everything to do with the ceremonies of life. When the kettle boiled, he poured, and the steam rose. He put mine beside my empty coffee mug and said, "Careful. Hot."

"You always say that."

"You always burn your tongue."

I took a sip. Burned my tongue.

He sat with his hand on the mug in front of him.

Except it wasn't blue.

Somewhere between the kettle and our conversation, we'd switched cups. The white cup sat by his hand. The blue one was between mine. We both noticed at the same time.

He stared at our cups. Then at me. "Did we just—"

"Switch cups," I said.

Somehow, we'd broken a law as reliable as gravity.

"Should we switch them back?" His voice caught on the word *back*.

"I already burned my tongue," I said. "Might as well commit to the chaos."

"But my cup—" He lifted the white one slightly, as if testing its weight.

"Drink the tea."

He took a sip.

"It tastes fine," he said.

"Shocking."

"But it feels wrong."

"That's your brain being weird about routines."

"My brain is very invested in my cup."

I didn't tell him, but knowing I was drinking from his blue mug felt strange. "Tell your tea we're living dangerously now."

CHAPTER 14

Sunday, June 14

Paul had printed things. I knew it was serious. He printed things when a problem had graduated from something he could hold in his head to something that required a physical record. The stack on the kitchen table was an inch thick. Insurance documents. Benefit summaries. A spreadsheet he had made himself. A printed webpage about SSDI eligibility with three paragraphs highlighted in yellow.

He had been at this since before I got up.

I stood in the doorway and looked at the stack. I wanted to avoid going in, but I'd run out of excuses.

"Sit down," he said eagerly. His voice carried the register of a man who had organized the facts and needed a witness.

I sat down.

He turned the spreadsheet to face me.

"Okay," he said. "Here's where we are."

The abdominal cramp arrived about ninety seconds later. Of course it did. Because the body has opinions and perfectly imperfect timing. It started low and wide, the kind of pain that announced itself as a situation rather than a passing inconvenience. I shifted in my chair.

Paul was explaining the difference between our current health plan and Medicare supplemental coverage, moving his pen along a column of numbers. I was nodding in the way that meant I was present and tracking, while simultaneously conducting an internal negotiation with my digestive system.

The negotiation was not going well.

"The deductible resets in January," Paul said. "Which means between now and December we're on the hook for..."

"Excuse me," I said.

I made it to the bathroom with a margin of dignity I would not describe as comfortable.

Constipation, incontinence, and cramping were not topics found in the inspirational literature about Parkinson's. The brochures in Dr. Patel's office, with their photographs of people smiling beside bicycles, did not educate me. I had learned the hard way...on the toilet. It was, as a subject, absent from polite conversation. It was present, however, with considerable enthusiasm in my lower abdomen.

I sat on the toilet and waited.

Paul's voice carried from the kitchen with the steady persistence of a man who had prepared a speech.

"—and the co-pay structure changes if I move you to a supplemental plan. Of course, that plan has a higher premium, so the question is whether we're better off with the lower premium and higher out-of-pocket or higher premium with better coverage."

The question, I thought, *is whether I will survive the next ten minutes.*

The cramps came in waves, the way they always did, arriving and receding...arriving again with the regularity of something that had nothing to do with bowel regularity. I pressed my palms against my thighs and breathed the way the physical therapist had taught me — not that she had taught me it for this application. It was a breathing technique for surviving dystonia's cramping pain without screaming in the middle of the night. But breath was breath.

Paul's lecture continued, "—the neurologist visits are going to be every three months or so, and at our current tier that's a hundred and forty dollars per visit after deductible, times four visits per year—"

I did the math automatically. *Five hundred and sixty dollars. Per year. For one doctor.*

The cramping eased slightly and then reconsidered. I shifted my weight.

"Levodopa is manageable. But if we get into other medications, we're looking at—"

He paused. I heard paper being moved.

"Joy?"

"Still here," I called.

"Okay." Papers shuffled. "So, if we look at the newer extended release, which Dr. Patel mentioned as a possibility, we're potentially at three hundred a month with our current coverage. That's before any add-ons."

Three hundred a month. I calculated: *thirty-six hundred a year just in medication. Inadequate medication, according to Dr. Patel,*

I assume adequate medicine would cost a kidney. If there is one.

Another wave arrived. I gripped the edge of the vanity with one hand and waited it out, thinking about the spreadsheet on the kitchen table. Paul's plan was this...finances...a fix within his reach. *He can't slow the progression or restore my brain. He can't remake the future into the one we planned. But he can build a spreadsheet.*

"—the disability timeline is the piece with the most variables."

I called out, "Paul."

"Yeah?"

"How long have you been working on this?"

A longer pause. "A couple of months."

I looked at the wall above the towel rack. There was a small water stain near the ceiling I hadn't noticed before, pale brown, roughly the shape of something that didn't resolve into anything. I looked at it for a moment.

"Okay," I said. "Keep going."

"—so, the documentation piece is important because the adjudicators look for a consistent medical record. Dr. Patel's notes will help, but we should also keep a symptom log. Daily if possible. Time of day, severity, what affected function and how."

A symptoms log? Oh crap. Another way to identify myself.

"—and the house modifications are something we should think about before we need them rather than after. The bathroom needs modifying."

I am, at this moment, producing material for the log, whether I want to or not.

"—grab bars, possibly a raised seat; the threshold between the bedroom and the hall is a tripping hazard—"

The cramp passed. Fully, with the exhaust of something that had made its point. I sat for another moment in the quiet of a bathroom that had returned to being an ordinary room...except for the smell.

"—the steps outside are a long-term question. I think I could build a ramp. It'll look better than those steps."

A raised toilet seat, I thought. *He'll research those. He'll find the one with the optimal angle and the correct load rating, and he'll install it. He won't say a word about what it means that we need one.*

I stood. Washed my hands. Looked at my reflection briefly and looked away.

"—so, the total picture, if I'm conservative—"

I came back down the hall and sat back down at the table.

Paul looked up. Looked at me with the quick assessment he had developed over the last year, the one that checked several things at once without appearing to check anything. Whatever he found, he didn't say.

I said, "Where were we?"

He found his place on the spreadsheet with his pen. "We can afford this." He set the pen down. Looked at me directly. "Are you okay?"

"I'm fine."

He held the look for a moment. The look that meant he knew *fine* was an operational term in our household with a flexible relationship to its dictionary definition.

"Okay," he said. He picked the pen back up.

"Paul."

He looked up again.

"You've been at this since six," I said.

"I know."

"On a Saturday."

"I needed to understand what we're dealing with. I needed to see the numbers."

"Show me the conservative estimate," I said.

He turned the spreadsheet back toward me, and we sat at the kitchen table and looked at the numbers together. The numbers were not good, but we looked at them anyway because talking about finances was doable.

CHAPTER 15

Friday, July 10

Paul stood and carried his blue cup to the sink. He dumped a full cup of coffee, rinsed it, rotating it under the stream of water. He placed it in the dish rack at an angle. He adjusted it, just a fraction. Then another.

"Paul."

"Hm?"

"What are you doing?"

"Making sure it drains properly." He turned the mug two degrees to the left. "If it dries wrong, water pools at the base."

"Gravity will handle it."

"Not if the angle is wrong."

He leaned in and adjusted it again.

"Paul."

He blinked. Looked at his hand as if he'd forgotten it was attached to him.

"The cup's fine," I said.

He pulled his hand away and came back to the table. "I'm really stressed about taking the lead on this project." He said after a moment.

"Mr. Richards accepted your report. Liked it enough to give you the lead."

"True."

"You want to do the project?"

"Richards also wants me to keep up with my current work."

The bitterness in his voice was new. Paul rarely complained about work. He believed in putting his head down and doing the job.

"Can you say no?"

He laughed without humor. "And watch the promotion go to Peter, who'll say yes because he doesn't have a sick wife to worry about."

His words stung.

"I'm sorry." Paul got up and walked over to me. His hands found my shoulders. "Joy, I'm sorry. That came out all wrong."

"I'm just stressed." He pulled me against him. "I'm worried. And when I'm worried, I say stupid things."

I pressed my face into his shoulder.

"You're not a burden," he said. I nodded against his chest.

He kissed my forehead. "I'm sorry."

"I know you need this promotion."

"And I know you need me here." His voice became soft. "We'll figure it out."

I nodded. But doubt crept in. "Paul, you really should consider taking the project."

"We just talked about this last night."

"I know. But I also know you need it. For your career."

"What I need," he said firmly, "is to be here. With you. We'll make it work, even without the promotion."

"But—"

"But nothing. I'd have to work a lot. Be gone for days, maybe a couple of weeks." He shook his head. "You need me here."

"You could commute. It's not far."

"You know that's not how Richards works. Once a project gets going, it's all hours."

"I can manage."

"Like you managed when you fell in the parking lot?"

What he said hurt because it confirmed what I'd feared: I was becoming Paul's burden.

"I'll be more careful," I said.

Paul's eyes moved to my hand, to the window, then back to my face. "I'll figure it out," he said. "I always do."

"I've never seen you so stressed."

"I know. It's just...I want to make sure we're ready. I can modify the house. Research the best doctors and the latest treatments and—"

His voice cracked. "I can do something. I'm not going to just sit here and watch you deteriorate while I do nothing."

"You're doing everything right," I said.

"But that's the problem. I can't find the right way to deal with this."

"There is no right way."

"There has to be." He said it with such conviction, such desperate need to believe it, that my heart broke a little. "If I just—if we just follow the plan."

"What plan, Paul?"

He didn't answer. He pulled me against him—hard, desperate, like he was trying to hold us both together.

"I don't have a plan," he breathed into my hair. "I don't know how to protect you from this. I don't know how to watch you get worse."

He still held me. "I'm supposed to know. I'm supposed to have answers."

"You're supposed to be human. That's all."

"I'm terrified," he finally said. "Of losing you. Of failing you. What if something happens and I'm not able to take care of you? Or be enough?"

"You're enough," I said.

He pulled back to look at my face. "I love you. You know that, right? Even when I'm being an idiot about promotions and saying terrible things?"

"I know."

"Good. Because I do. Love you. So much."

He kissed me—gentle, careful, like I might break. Then he rested his forehead against mine.

I knew Paul. His inability to fix the problem...me... would feel like failure to Paul.

CHAPTER 16

Saturday, July 11

Once we decided he should take the lead on the project, Paul went right to work — emerging from his office only to refill his coffee and apologize for "just one more hour" that turned into three.

"Paul? It's almost seven." I was standing at his office door.

He flinched and looked up. His eyes took a second to settle on my face. "Is it?" He closed his eyes. "God. Sorry." His gaze dropped back to the monitor. "I just need to finish this section."

"We had plans."

His fingers paused above the keys. Then they started again.

"The movie," I said. "The one I circled on the calendar."

He frowned at the screen, scrolling. The light from the monitor painted his cheekbones blue.

"I'm sorry, Joy. This project. Can we watch a movie when I get back?"

Two weeks.

I kept my hand on the doorframe so it wouldn't dance. My thumb pressed into my palm until it hurt. "Sure," I said. "No problem."

Paul nodded without looking up, as if agreement had been the only obstacle.

I stepped into the room. The air smelled like garlic had a date with chocolate. Paper covered the corner of his desk in neat piles, each stack squared. On the wall, the calendar hung. Tonight was circled in red.

Paul's eyes stayed on the screen.

"It's the movie we've been talking about for weeks," I said.

He made a small sound that could have been a sigh. Then he said, "I'll make it up to you." His hands kept typing.

I waited for him to swivel in his chair and look at me.

He did not.

I walked to the calendar and put my finger on the red circle. My handwriting looked childish next to his printed schedules and numbered deadlines. "It's a shame we'll miss it."

He glanced over, quick as a mirror check while driving, and returned to the screen. "Yes," he said. "It is. But we'll catch a different one."

I let my hand fall. The tremor started as a small vibration in my fingers.

Paul's gaze flicked down. "You need your next dose?" he asked.

"I already took it."

He adjusted his glasses with the knuckle of his index finger and looked back at the screen.

I stood there long enough to feel myself growing impatient.

A movie trailer's song reached us from the living room TV. I had left it on earlier to keep the house from feeling empty. A couple laughed on-screen. A door slammed. Music swelled.

Paul pressed his palms against his forehead. "The TV is too loud."

I turned and walked away before I said something I couldn't take back.

In the bedroom, I changed into pajamas, even though it was early. My heavy jeans lay in a heap beside the bed. I looked at them and left them where they were — *not worth the effort.* I sat on the edge of the mattress and flexed my right hand until the tremor eased.

On the nightstand, my phone lit up. Unknown number. I watched it until the screen went dark.

Then it lit again.

Same number.

I answered. "Hello?"

"Mrs. Anderson? This is Marcus, from the gym."

Why would he call me?

"Hi," I said.

"I need you to come in on Monday," he said. "Before your session. There's something we need to discuss."

My fingers tightened around the phone. "Is everything okay?"

"I'd rather talk in person," Marcus said.

"What is this about?"

In the silence of his pause, I heard metal clank and someone laughing.

"It's nothing to worry about," he said.

"I'll be in," I said. "Around eleven."

"Thank you. Good night."

The call ended.

I lowered the phone onto the nightstand. My right hand kept moving, as if my body hadn't received the message that the call was over or understood that I'd already taken the levodopa.

From down the hall, Paul's chair shifted.

I went back to his door. He hadn't moved. A half-full coffee cup sat by his keyboard — not his blue mug, the one he always used, but a clear glass one. He picked it up and held it loosely, drank without looking at it, and set it down. The base made a soft click. He nudged it a fraction of an inch.

"Paul," I said.

He looked up. His expression softened when he saw my face. Then his gaze drifted back to the screen.

"I got a call," I said.

"From work?"

What is he talking about? I haven't worked in years.

"From the gym."

That pulled him back. His eyebrows lifted.

"Marcus," I said. "He wants to meet on Monday. Before my session."

Paul's eyes moved to my right hand, then to my face. "Your meds not kicking in? You should call Dr. Patel."

"I'm alright. More concerned about the gym."

"Did something happen?" he asked.

"No," I said. "Not that I know of."

He stood and reached for my arm. His hand hovered, then landed lightly above my elbow. He used to grab my arm firmly — without thinking.

"You're okay," he said.

Is he telling me? Or himself.

"I think it's about when I fell," I said. "I might lose my membership."

He nodded once. He rubbed his thumb against my sleeve in a small, repetitive motion. Then he stopped himself. "That would be terrible."

"I like going there. It gives me something to do. I hate just sitting here in the house."

"We will handle it," he said. "There are other gyms." He was already back at his desk.

I nodded.

"I need to finish this," he said.

"I know."

After a few minutes, I gave up and walked to the living room alone. I turned off the TV. The sudden quiet made the house feel larger.

I stood at the window. Cars drove past. The sun was still up, but I wished it wasn't.

At seven-fifteen, my phone buzzed with a calendar reminder.

MOVIE — JOY + PAUL

I stared at the words until my eyes blurred. My thumb hovered. Then I deleted the alert.

In the kitchen, I opened the cabinet for a glass. My eyes went to the gallon jug on the counter.

I filled the glass from the tap, lifted it to my mouth and drank.

The water tasted like water.

I poured it out, refilled it from the jug, and drank that instead.

Well, guess the water's not too bad. I didn't fall to the floor like a dying bug.

From his office, Paul called, "Joy?"

"Yes."

"I'm going to work a little longer. Do you want tea?"

"Yes," I said. "Tea sounds good."

He didn't come out right away. I stood waiting for the water to boil.

Paul came in, opened the cabinet, and took down two cups: his blue one and my white one. He placed them side by side, handles facing out.

He caught me watching. "What?"

"Nothing."

He said, "Are you alright? Do you need anything? I could make you a snack."

"No thanks," I said. "Tea is good."

He opened the drawer for the tea bags, selected chamomile, and placed one in each cup.

Chamomile. Good choice. I need to relax.

"We don't have popcorn anyway," he said, as if the movie could still be negotiated. "And the previews are always loud."

I said nothing.

The kettle began to vibrate. Steam curled from the spout. Paul stood with his shoulders tense. When the whistle blew, he flinched.

He poured the water and set the kettle down. "Careful," he said, sliding my cup toward me. "It's hot."

I took it. The ceramic warmed my palms. My hand shook enough that the liquid sloshed a little.

Paul reached out to grab it, then stopped himself. "I will make this up to you," he said.

I nodded. "I know."

He took a sip and winced. "Too hot."

"You warned me."

He smiled. His eyes drifted back toward the hallway, toward his office. "Do you want me to stop?"

The question surprised me. My grip tightened on the mug. "Honestly, yes."

He hesitated. The kettle clicked as it cooled. Paul looked disappointed. "I can't tonight," he said. "I'm sorry."

I blew on my tea.

"I won't be too late," he said.

"I'm going to bed."

He nodded. "I'll come in when I'm done."

I carried my cup to the sink and poured the tea out. I rinsed the cup and placed it in the rack. It landed crooked. I didn't fix it. Paul noticed.

"Good night," he said. "Don't be angry. I need to work."

"Good night."

I left him standing in the kitchen with his tea and his focus.

In the bedroom, I lay on my back and stared at the slowly turning ceiling fan as it cut the air into even pieces.

The movie started without us.

CHAPTER 17

Saturday, July 11

I was in bed long enough for the sun to go down. I turned onto my side and pressed my knees together, relaxing, until my body stopped buzzing. The sheets were cool. I focused on the sound of the fan, counting the blades as they passed the light. I switched off the light by the bed.

From the hallway came the scrape of Paul's chair.

The bedroom door opened a few inches. Light spilled across the floor, stopping at the edge of the mattress.

"Are you asleep?" he asked.

"Yes," I said.

I heard him take a slow breath, as if he were about to say something else. The door closed.

I stared into the darkness until my eyes adjusted. The ceiling fan blurred into a circle. Somewhere outside, a neighbor laughed. When I fell asleep, I dreamed of water rising to a line etched inside a tea kettle, stopping just short of where it was supposed to be. No matter how much water I added, the kettle never filled.

CHAPTER 18

Monday, July 13

Morning light cut through the window and landed on the hall floor in a clean rectangle. Paul's office door was open. His voice carried from inside, clipped and professional. He was on the phone.

"Right. I understand the timeline."

I went to the kitchen for coffee.

Paul's cup is still on the hook. Where's mine?

I filled my spare cup halfway.

"I can be on-site tomorrow evening," Paul said. "Full assessment...That's right. Preliminary plan in ten to twelve days."

Tomorrow. I thought he'd be home for a few more days. I should make him a nice dinner. Make up for being selfish last night.

I took a sip. The coffee was too hot. My hand jerked, and the liquid sloshed over the rim, hitting my fingers. I leaned over the sink, spitting the mouthful out while shaking it off my hand. I turned on the cold water and held my fingers under it. The sting dulled.

"No, that will not be a problem," Paul said. "My wife will be fine."

I shut off the water and grabbed a towel. Coffee dripped down the front of the cabinet. I wiped it up and added cream to what was left in the mug. The coffee turned pale...and cold.

"Yes, I reviewed the file," Paul said.

I left my cup where it was and walked into his office.

He sat at his desk with his phone pressed to his ear. He smiled when he saw me and pointed to the couch as if I was a visitor who had arrived during office hours.

"Absolutely," Paul said.

He ended the call and turned to me, his face shifting as he recalibrated.

"Morning," I said.

"You're up early."

He sat on the couch beside me and reached for my feet, lifting them into his lap. His hands were warm. He pressed his thumbs into my arches.

"Your feet are cold," he said.

His eyes drifted to the doorway. His thumbs kept moving, but I could feel his attention splitting.

"What are you worried about?" he asked.

Paul seems different. Slower. Older.

"I'm just tired," I said. "Still waking up."

"Did you sleep?"

"Enough." I looked at his face. "Did you?"

"I got up early." His hands slowed. Then he stopped rubbing my feet.

"What was the call about?" I asked.

"They need me on-site," he said. "I will pack now and leave this morning."

"Today?"

"They are putting me up in a hotel." He glanced at his watch. "It makes more sense."

I followed his gaze to the side table.

He has my cup.

Paul lifted it and took a sip.

I stared.

"Is that my white cup?" I asked.

He looked at it as if it had just appeared in his hand. "Is it?"

He frowned. "I just grabbed."

"Is this a special occasion?" I asked.

He said, "I was focused on getting ready. Got the wrong cup."

"That much is clear." I pulled my feet from his lap and laughed. "Drink from it. Live dangerously. Next, you will be using the good towels."

"We have good towels?"

"The white ones. You said they were only for guests."

He said, "I've been using those all week."

"I know." I laughed harder. "And last week too."

I took the cup from his hands and tasted the coffee. It was sweet to the point of surrendering.

"This is terrible," I said.

"I like it that way."

I made a face. "This is a beverage that gave up."

He almost smiled.

"So, you will be gone for two weeks?" I asked.

"Could be less," he said. "Depends."

He took off his glasses. "You will be okay. You have enough medication. I left phone numbers on the fridge."

"Fine," I said.

He looked at me for a moment. Then he stood. "I need to pack."

I stayed on the couch, drinking his sweet coffee.

Twenty-five minutes later, Paul came into the office with his suitcase. He'd changed into khakis and a polo shirt.

"All set," he said. "I'll call you once I'm settled."

I followed him to the door. We stood in the entryway. He set down his suitcase and pulled me into an embrace. His arms were stiff and awkward.

Is something wrong with him?

I pulled away from him.

"Paul. I'm sorry about last night."

"What happened last night?" He smiled and gave me a proper hug.

"Be safe," I said into his shoulder.

"It's just two weeks. You can call me if you need something."

"I know."

He patted his pockets. Frowned. "Where are my keys?"

I pointed at his other hand.

He looked down, surprised to find them there.

"Right. Of course." He laughed, but it came out thin. "Rushing around so much, I'm liable to forget my own feet."

Everyone forgets things when they're stressed. Everyone pats their pockets looking for keys they're already holding. It doesn't mean anything.

"I'll miss you," he said.

"Love you more," I answered.

He kissed my forehead. Picked up his suitcase. Opened the door.

"Paul."

He turned back.

"I do love you," I said.

"I love you too."

The door closed behind him.

I watched him through the window.

His hands were on the steering wheel. Then his forehead dropped forward until it touched his knuckles.

His shoulders began to shake.

I wanted to run outside. Wanted to tap on the window and make him look at me. I wanted to hold him the way he'd so often held me when I cried in pain from dystonia. But I knew my body wouldn't move fast enough. By the time I reached the door, he would have already been pulling away.

I stood there with my palm flat against the window and watched Paul fall apart in the driveway.

He wiped his face with both hands. Then he sat up straight. Checked the rearview mirror. Put the car in reverse.

He didn't look back at the house.

The car backed out of the driveway and disappeared down the street.

I stayed at the window long after he was gone, my hand still pressed against the glass, my reflection staring back at me.

CHAPTER 19

Monday, July 13

Our house inhaled silence. The clock said 10:17.

I have two weeks.

I took my second pill of the day, quite a bit early. I grabbed my keys and purse, leaving before the silence convinced me to stay.

The grocery store was nearly empty. A woman was partially blocking an aisle, talking into her phone, laughing. A man stood at the cooler, staring at the milk.

I walked through the aisles without a list. I chose a can of soup and a box of crackers. I put a case of water in the cart.

In the meat section, I stopped. Five packs of liver sat on the shelf. *I don't eat liver. Paul does.*

I put all five in the cart and pushed on.

At the checkout, a young man scanned the water, crackers, soup, and the air freshener. Then he picked up the first pack of liver. Then the second. He slowed down at the third one. By the fourth, he looked up.

"Stocking up?" he asked.

"Preparing for the apocalypse," I said, smiling as if eating liver when the world ends was totally normal.

He didn't smile as he read the total to me.

My hands fumbled for my wallet and I dropped it.

Of course.

I bent to reach it and felt the shift before it happened. I caught myself on the counter and stayed there until my feet decided my being vertical was a good idea.

The man came around and handed me my wallet.

"Thanks," I said.

I swiped the card the wrong way. Then I pulled it out before the beep.

Slow down. It's not like you have anything else to do today.

"You have to wait," he said.

"Sorry," I said. "The machine and I are in a complicated relationship. It wants commitment. I keep swiping left."

He laughed. "That's good," he said. "I'm using that."

"It's yours. Free of charge."

The machine finally accepted my card.

"There we go," I said. "My hands shake, but my credit's solid."

He glanced at my hands, then away quickly.

"I have Parkinson's. I'm a shaky mess."

"Oh."

"What's your excuse?" I asked. "For not laughing at my joke."

He blinked. "I thought you were serious."

"I might be," I said.

He handed me the receipt and wished me a nice day, as if he were reading from a script.

Outside, the sun felt too bright. The parking lot stretched in every direction, full of cars belonging to people who had somewhere to be or someone to get back to. I loaded the bags into the trunk.

By the time I closed the trunk, my hands were steady.

Parkinson's makes me count victories in minutes. Twenty minutes of steady hands. Two hours until my next pill. Fourteen days before Paul comes home. Fourteen days is a lot of minutes.

CHAPTER 20
Monday, July 13

The gym doors sighed open. Pine cleaner, sharp and artificial, tried to cover sweat and old rubber. *Marcus must have switched products.*

The floor felt sticky under my shoes. I'd walked this floor for three years. I knew where the rubber seams were. Where the concrete showed through worn patches and weight plates had left permanent dark circles like rust-colored ghosts.

Weights clanged somewhere behind me. A man on the bench press grunted—deep, guttural sounds like he was giving birth. Each rep was louder than the last. The whole gym, apparently, was his witness.

At the cable machine, I rested my fingers on the cold metal handle. Its texture pressed into my palm, familiar as a handshake. *Probably the last time I'll touch this.* I let go.

In the mirror wall, I caught my reflection. I looked fine...hair pulled back, shoulders straight.

Marcus's office door was open. He sat behind his desk, staring at his computer as if it had personally betrayed him. I knocked on the doorframe.

He looked up and gestured to the chair. "Joy. Thanks for coming in."

"This is where you fire me, right?"

"We're not firing you."

"Terminating my membership."

"—modifying our requirements." He slid a piece of paper across the desk as if he were presenting evidence at trial. "Dr. Patel's note isn't sufficient."

I looked at the paper. It was my medical clearance, the one Dr. Patel had written, saying I could exercise with modifications.

"How's it insufficient?"

"It approves some activities and limits others. My boss requires unrestricted clearance."

Unrestricted.

I let the word sit there a moment before I responded. "Marcus, I have Parkinson's disease. The restrictions are kind of built in. Factory settings."

He didn't smile. I'm pretty sure his face was set to neutral at birth.

He said, "I understand that."

"Do you need me to get a note from God? Because he probably has activity restrictions for people with degenerative neurological conditions. No smiting, for instance. Too much arm repetition."

Nothing. Not even a flicker. This man is a black hole.

"Our insurance requires unrestricted medical clearance for all members." He folded his hands on the desk. "If you can get that from Dr. Patel, we'd be happy to reinstate your membership."

"And if I can't?"

"Then I can't let you back on the floor."

"Can I see the letter?" I asked. "The one from your insurance?"

He hesitated. "Internal policy."

"So, there's a policy that excludes people with disabilities."

"I wouldn't phrase it that way."

"How would you phrase it?"

He shifted in his chair. "We have to protect the gym from liability."

"Marcus, I fell in the lot weeks ago. Nobody sued you."

"That's different."

"How?"

"You weren't technically on gym property."

I stared at him. "I was ten feet from your door."

"The parking lot is separately insured."

"You're worried I'll fall inside instead of outside?"

"I'm just following policy."

"Right. Can I get a copy of the internal policy? The one that says people with Parkinson's can't work out?"

"It doesn't say that specifically."

"But it requires unrestricted clearance, which I can't get. You're excluding me because of my disability."

I walked out before he could respond.

CHAPTER 21

Monday, July 13

After the gym, I went home and sat in the driveway without getting out. Across the street, Mrs. Henderson's front door was open. A blue sedan sat in her driveway that I didn't recognize.

A woman came out of Mrs. Henderson's home with a cardboard box. She placed it in the trunk, went back inside, and returned with another. Then another.

Is Mrs. Henderson moving?

On her fourth trip, she looked straight at me. We held eye contact across the street. I got out of my car and walked over. The woman had already gone back inside. Through the open door, I could see the hallway. It was filled with labeled boxes: kitchen, bedroom, living room. The house smelled of lemon cleaner. I knocked.

A woman appeared with another box in her arms. Up close, she had Mrs. Henderson's facial features but none of her softness.

"Yes?" she said.

"I'm Joy," I said. "From across the street."

She nodded. "Mom mentioned you."

"Is Mrs. Henderson alright?" I asked.

"She's being admitted to a memory care facility."

"When?"

"Today." She set the box down. "She has dementia," the daughter said, closing a chapter.

"How long?" I asked. "How long has she had dementia?"

"Over a year." She rubbed her forehead. "She wouldn't accept help."

"Can I visit her?" I asked.

"No," the answer came fast. "She gets confused by visitors."

I looked past her into the house, at the boxes that held Mrs. Henderson's life.

She followed my gaze. "I need to finish packing."

The door closed. The blue sedan sat in the driveway, trunk still open. The boxes inside were stacked flush against each other, labels facing out, each one the same size.

A hawk sat on a tree at the edge of Mrs. Henderson's yard. I watched it until it flew. I crossed back to our house.

In a box labeled JOY, what would fit? What wouldn't I pack at all?

CHAPTER 22

Tuesday, July 14

I'd been awake since before midnight. Not worrying. Just awake. I stared at the ceiling while listening to the house creak and crack. I counted the drips from the kitchen faucet. At midnight, I'd sent Paul a message: "Everything okay?"

He always called when he traveled — three times a day minimum: morning coffee, lunch break, before bed. Years of business trips, and he'd never once let a day pass without checking in, repeatedly.

Not after what happened in Phoenix.

Until yesterday.

I'd turned the phone face down after sending the text, telling myself I wasn't the kind of person who needed constant reassurance. But when the phone chirped at 3:17 in the morning, I grabbed my phone so fast that I nearly launched it across the room.

"Sorry. Been busy. Fell asleep".

I stared at the screen. Waiting for more.

"Long day. Will call tonight."

There must be more.

"Love you."

I read the message three times because it felt like it had been typed between elevator floors.

He's tired. You're tired.

But Paul isn't tired. Paul is busy. There's a difference.

I put the phone down.

Don't look at it again.

I picked it up and read, "Will call tonight."

The last time he'd traveled for a big project — Houston — he'd called me from the airport, then from the hotel, then after his first meeting because the client had said something funny and Paul wanted to tell me about it. Then he called me at dinner so I could help him choose between the salmon and steak.

He said, "I need your expertise."

"Get the salmon."

"You always say that."

"Because you always want the steak and then complain about how heavy it is."

He'd gotten the salmon and called me afterwards to say I was right. Told me he loved me before hanging up.

There used to be three calls in one evening. Now I get text messages.

I pressed my fist against my thigh and focused on the pressure.

He's not avoiding me He's just busy.

But he's never been too busy for a call.

Not after Phoenix.

That was three years ago — a five-day sustainable building conference. During that trip, he'd stopped calling. I'd called the hotel. They'd confirmed he was checked in. I'd called his cell and my call went straight to voicemail. I called Mr. Richards, who assured me that Paul was fine. By day five, I'd been ready to call the police.

He'd walked through the door on the sixth day as if nothing had happened. When I asked why I hadn't heard from him, he said: "Thinking."

We'd fought. Badly.

I told him he couldn't just disappear and make me believe something terrible had happened. He apologized and said he'd gotten overwhelmed. At first, he claimed the conference had been intense. So, he needed space to process, had turned his phone off and lost track of time.

But he said, "It will never happen again."

And it hadn't.

Until now.

This isn't Phoenix. He's texting. He said he'll call.

But the shape of it felt the same: the silence, the distance, the clipped words.

When Paul finally explained Phoenix, he'd said: "I needed to figure out if I can do it. If I'm strong enough."

"Do what?"

"Stay. Watch you get worse. Be the person who would push your wheelchair when you can't walk anymore."

He'd held me then, promising he would always be here, and would never make me worry again.

That was before the tremors got worse. Before I started falling. Before the gym.

I put the phone face down on the nightstand.

I breathed in and counted to four. Breathed out and counted to four.

The house creaked. The faucet dripped. Outside, a car passed, and its headlights moved across the ceiling.

I lay there in the dark and let the silence fill in around me the way water fills the shape of whatever holds it.

I won't call him. I won't call.

CHAPTER 23

Tuesday, July 14

Stiffness pushed me to get up at five. I sat at the kitchen table, watching the faucet drip. It had no rhythm or pattern. The water escaped whenever gravity won. I considered whether a hammer counted as a legitimate plumbing tool, which seemed like the kind of logic Paul would approve of.

If he were here.

He isn't.

So, the faucet kept dripping, and I kept not fixing it, and we were both very committed to our dysfunction.

Dirty dishes were in the sink: a frying pan with dried egg and two plates. My white coffee cup was on the counter, with a thin ring of dried coffee marking the base.

He used my coffee cup.

Paul was superstitious about his blue coffee mug. Said his cup was good luck. He believed that his best ideas came with the first sip from that cup. When we moved to this house, he packed the blue cup first. Before the coffee maker, the plates, or anything else. Wrapped it in a dish towel and carried it in his jacket pocket during the drive.

"Priorities, Joy. A man needs his luck and his memories."

I laughed and told him he was ridiculous.

"Ridiculously in love with you," he said.

The cup doesn't mean anything.

Except Paul always used the blue one. Even in Phoenix. The morning after he got back, he said, "I forgot my cup. Left it in the hotel room."

"Call the hotel. Have them ship it."

"It's not the same," he said. "I broke the pattern."

FedEx brought the cup home. It arrived in bubble wrap.

It's a cup. Not a message. Not a sign. Just a cup.

Except it wasn't just a cup anymore.

He used my cup. That means something.

I liked the white cup because it was heavier than it looked.

He used my cup because he was thinking about missing me. You're reading too much into this.

My fingers rubbed the edge of the mug. I considered washing it and pretending nothing had shifted. Instead, I picked it up, carried my cup to the cabinet and shoved it to the back — unwashed. I took Paul's blue cup off the hook and slid it beside my own. I closed the cupboard door and turned away.

Drip. Drip.

I took my medication with bottled water. Swallowed the little white pill and made a face at the plastic aftertaste.

The clock said 8:15. Forty-five minutes until the support group meeting.

Drip.

At least I'll have something to do that isn't staring at cups and counting drips like a Victorian shut-in.

CHAPTER 24

Tuesday, July 14

The support group met in a room that smelled like death was taking its time.

Room 107...easily identifiable by the burned coffee.

Folding chairs were arranged in a circle as if we were about to summon something, which I supposed we were — a cure, maybe, or at least the willingness to get through another week without jumping off a bridge.

The handwritten sign on the door read: "Parkinson's Support Group - Tuesdays 9am - All Welcome!"

The exclamation point is a lie. Nothing about Parkinson's warrants an exclamation point. Maybe an ellipsis. Definitely a question mark.

I stood in the doorway, hand on the frame, feeling my fingers do their involuntary dance against the wood. The same fingers that used to move across piano keys without thinking and marked student papers. The hand that had started writing a book, back when my brain and hand were still on speaking terms.

About a year ago, I'd made it through three bars of *Silent Night* before my fingers refused to take on the chorus. Paul had looked up from his book, and I'd seen it on his face — that flicker of recognition that something else had been lost. He'd gone back to reading. I gave up, closed the piano lid, and turned on the TV.

I shouldn't be here. Go home and sit in front of the TV like a normal person having a breakdown.

"Are you coming in or planning to haunt the doorway?"

Rebecca was holding two Styrofoam cups of what might have been coffee in a former life.

"Haunting seemed safer," I said.

"It's not that bad." She handed me one of the cups. "Well, the coffee is that bad. But there are cookies."

"What kind?"

"The pretty ones that come wrapped in plastic."

"So, they're perfect for depression."

"With rainbow sprinkles." She smiled. "Come on. The first time might be rough. After that, it's just regular terrible."

I followed her into the room.

Twelve people had arranged themselves around the circle. Their ages ranged from what looked like late forties to a man who might have been ninety.

Three people had visible tremors. Two had the mask-like facial expression I recognized from my neurologist's waiting room. One woman sat perfectly still in a way that suggested stillness required significant effort. A younger man — maybe forty — sat slumped in his wheelchair, his head tilted at an angle his neck muscles couldn't quite correct. His eyes tracked us as we entered, bright and alert in a body that had stopped cooperating.

I forced myself to look at his face instead of his curled hands, but the image stayed burned in my peripheral vision. I flicked my fingers, driving the tremor away.

Most of the other people looked normal. There was a woman in running shoes and athletic gear. A man scrolled through his phone with only the slightest tremor. A few people were talking and laughing.

Rebecca led me to two empty chairs beside an older woman who was knitting something that might have been a scarf or might have been a cry for help. It was hard to tell with the color choices and the sheer ambition involved.

Rebecca said, "Joy, this is Diane."

"Nice to meet you," I said, the way you say things you don't mean to people you didn't want to meet in a room that shouldn't exist.

A woman stood and moved to the center of the circle. She wore yoga pants and a sweatshirt that said "Parkinson's Warrior" in glittery letters that suggested someone meant well but understood nothing.

"I'm Linda," she said. "I facilitate. Which means I make sure we don't spend the whole hour complaining about neurologists."

"What if our neurologist deserves it?" one man asked.

"Gerald, I'll give you one minute. After that, take it to the Better Business Bureau." Linda smiled. "We have some new faces today. You know who you are. We're informal here. Just jump in and introduce yourself when you're ready. How's everyone doing this week?"

The woman in running shoes spoke first. "I'm Michelle. Diagnosed eight months ago. Stage one." She said it as if she were announcing a prison sentence. "Slight tremor in my hand. Some stiffness in my shoulder. That's it. That's all I have."

"That's all you have so far," Gerald said.

"Jesus, Gerald," Diane muttered.

"What? I'm only being honest. Stage one is the opening act. Wait till the second half."

Michelle's jaw tightened. "My neurologist says if I exercise regularly and manage stress, I might stay at stage one for years. Maybe a decade."

"And you believe him?" Gerald asked.

"I have to believe in something."

I shifted in my seat.

"I came because my husband doesn't get it," Michelle continued. "He keeps saying it's not that bad. That I'm overreacting." Her voice cracked. "But I can feel it. Every morning, it seems a little worse. And he wants me to pretend it's not happening."

I looked down at my coffee. The surface rippled.

Don't relate to her. Don't make this about solidarity.

"They all do," Diane said, not looking up from her knitting. "Husbands, wives, doctors. We do it too, if we're honest."

Rebecca said, "What do you mean?"

"Call it a tremor when we mean a decline. Call it a bad day when we mean it's getting worse. Try to be polite and say we're fine, when what we really want to do is scream."

A man across from me spoke next. "Martin. Week six post-DBS surgery." He touched his head where his hair was growing back over the surgical scars.

"Welcome back, Martin. We missed you," Linda said.

Another man said, "What's the verdict? Did it work?"

Martin said, "Still getting used to the settings. Too much one way, and I'll be twisting around so much a snake would be jealous. Too little, and the tremors hit. But I like it. I feel more like myself."

Diane asked, "How's the falling?" Diane looked at me. She said, "Martin used to fall a lot. The last time, what was it? In the grocery?"

Martin said, "By the banana display."

"What did the produce manager do?" Diane asked.

"Gave me a discount on bananas. He probably thought a banana tripped me."

Everyone laughed.

"Free bananas," Diane said. "That's what I call a win."

"They drilled into your brain?" Gerald asked. "Seems extreme."

"Gerald," Linda said, "we talked about this."

"I'm just saying. They put wires in your head and call it treatment. In my day, that was called science fiction."

"In your day," Diane said, "they also prescribed cocaine for headaches. Medical science evolves."

Gerald said, "I'm not that old, Diane."

Diane huffed, "Close enough."

Martin shrugged. "The tremor's better. But yeah, they drilled into my skull. Put a battery pack in my chest and wires in my head. Now I can negotiate my symptoms."

Gerald said, "How does it work? By a remote control?"

Martin said, "When you say it out loud, it does sound insane."

For a second I imagined myself on an operating table, skull open, some surgeon's hands inside my brain trying to fix what medication couldn't.

Would I still be me after that?

Remote-controlled brain. Is that where this is heading?

A woman beside Martin shifted forward — the one who sat perfectly still. Her voice was barely audible, breathy. "Elizabeth. Diagnosed six years ago. No tremor."

I blinked.

"Wait," I said. "You can have Parkinson's without a tremor?"

Linda said, "Not everyone with Parkinson's develops a tremor. Some have rigidity-dominant symptoms."

"But I thought—" I stopped.

"Parkinson's equals shaking?" Elizabeth's attempted smile didn't reach her eyes.

A man said, “I'm David. Elizabeth's son. She does yoga to help with her symptoms.”

“Did yoga help?” I asked. My voice came out steadier than I felt.

“Only in that it confirmed she can't touch her toes anymore. But Mom says she likes doing it.”

The room made sympathetic noises.

A younger woman — late forties, her left hand resting carefully on her lap — spoke next. “I'm Jennifer. Mostly I'm just tired. All the time. Like someone replaced my blood with cement.”

“Fatigue's a bitch,” Diane said.

“My kids think I'm lazy. My boss thinks I'm checked out. My husband bought me vitamins.” Jennifer’s laugh was hollow.

Linda said, “Vitamins might be a good idea. B-12 deficiency has been connected to Parkinson's and Parkinson's-related dementia.”

“Dementia. Like we don't have enough problems,” Diane said.

David said, “It's true. Mom's neurologist has her get B12 injections.”

A woman wearing a pink shirt said, “Better a shot than more pills.”

“I take sixteen pills a day,” Gerald said. “Not one of them is a vitamin.”

Diane looked at Gerald. “I bet they're all levodopa.”

“How'd you know?”

She said, “Could be the way you're moving.”

A woman beside Gerald — with a barely visible tremor — raised her hand. "I'm on four medications. Two of them are for side effects from the others. My pharmacist knows me by name now. We're basically dating."

A balding man, with a cane beside his knee, spoke up. "I'm Robert. I want to talk about sex."

The room fell silent.

Linda blinked. "Robert, I don't think that is an appropriate topic. We usually—"

"No one talks about it," Robert said. "But it's a problem. The medications mess with everything. Ropinirole made me hypersexual for months. I was flirting with my wife like I was a teenager. She thought I'd lost my mind."

"Had you?" Gerald asked.

"Probably. But it was the medication. Once they adjusted it, my libido disappeared entirely." He gestured vaguely. "And my wife doesn't know if it's the disease, the medication, or if I'm just not attracted to her anymore."

Gerald said, "Increased libido doesn't sound like a terrible side effect. My wife wouldn't mind if I were a bit younger. Come to think of it, the same goes for me."

"Have you talked to her about it?" Diane asked.

Gerald looked at Diane with his jaw dropped. "Who? My wife?"

"No, Tinkerbell. Of course, your wife. I just think some subjects should be discussed at home, but they're not. Like, maybe Robert should speak openly with his wife. Then we wouldn't end up in rabbit holes like this."

Robert said, "I'm sixty-five years old."

Diane set down her knitting. "And that's a bad excuse for not talking at home. You're talking about it now. In a room full of strangers. Maybe try talking to your wife."

"It's easier to talk here," Robert said.

I thought about Paul's face when I'd stopped mid-nocturne. He wasn't angry or sad. Just resigned. Like he was watching something die in real time and had already started grieving it.

The woman beside the man in a wheelchair touched her husband's shoulder. He made a sound, soft and unintelligible. She leaned close, listening, then looked at Robert. "Tom says the hardest part isn't losing the ability. It's watching me become his caregiver instead of his wife...Oh, my name is Sarah."

CHAPTER 25

Tuesday, July 14

I pressed my thumb into the side of my empty cup until it buckled and set it down quickly when I felt moisture.

"I don't know how to be both," Sarah continued, her voice cracking. "His wife and his caregiver. When I'm helping him dress, helping him eat, helping him use the bathroom — there's no romance in wiping someone's chin."

Tom made another sound: louder, sharper.

Sarah's hand moved to his. "I know. I'm sorry. I know you hate this, too."

I stared at Tom's curled hands in Sarah's capable ones. I imagined Paul's hands holding mine that way.

"I've tried five different medications," a woman said. "Each one was worse than the last. Dyskinesia. Hallucinations. Nausea. I gave up and started focusing on exercise instead."

"Does it help?" I asked.

"It's the only thing that helps. Medication manages symptoms. Exercise might slow progression. Insurance will only pay for pills, but not for gym memberships."

"My gym just kicked me out," I said.

The words came out before I could stop them. The room's eyes turned.

Shit. Why did I say that? I didn't come here to share. I came to observe.

"Liability concerns," I continued, my voice sharper than necessary. "I fell in their parking lot. Now I need unrestricted medical clearance, which I can't get, because—" I gestured at myself. "Parkinson's comes with restrictions."

"That's illegal," Martin said.

I said, "Probably. But fighting it costs money I don't have and energy I'm running out of. And honestly? I'm not into exercise. I only went because spending time at the gym made me feel normal."

My voice cracked on the last word. I pressed my lips together, forcing myself not to cry in front of these people.

"What stage are you at?" Linda asked.

"Dr. Patel says I'm probably stage three. But she doesn't like staging."

"I take it you have symptoms on both sides?" Linda said.

I nodded. "Both sides affected, but I'm still—"

Still what? Still functional? Still me?

"Does it get easier?" Michelle asked.

"I have no idea," I said. "I used to play the piano. I can't anymore. My husband suggested I try taking up watercolors instead. Something less precise. As if I can just trade one thing for another and call it even."

"What did you say?" Diane asked.

"Nothing. I went to the bedroom." I shook my head. "I mean, what is there to say when things fall apart or a body fails?"

"The coffee tastes like failure in this group," Gerald said. "That's why I keep coming back. It's familiar."

Rebecca said, "I came because I'm not alone here. Even Gerald is comforting."

Everyone, including Gerald, laughed.

"I didn't come here for comfort," I said. "I came because I needed to see." I stopped.

"See what?" Rebecca asked gently.

"That I'm not crazy. That I'm not the only one. That—" I took a deep breath. "That I'm not being dramatic about losing my gym membership. It's not just the gym. It's everything. I'm losing everything."

"Exactly," Michelle said quietly.

Gerald added, "That's the truth of it. Parkinson's won't stop stealing."

I said, "My husband thinks I should just accept it and move on. Adjust. And maybe he's right."

"Are you asking us or telling us?" Diane asked.

I looked at her scarf growing longer despite her tremor.

"I don't know," I said. "I don't know what I'm doing here."

Rebecca touched my arm.

I said, "From where I'm sitting, it looks like we're all just slowly falling apart and maybe pretending there's a plan."

Silence.

Diane's needles stopped clicking. "Sixteen years ago," she said, "I was a concert violinist. Session work mostly, but some solo performances. Good enough to make a living."

She held up her hands. Both tremoring visibly.

"These hands played Carnegie Hall twice. Now they can barely hold knitting needles. Some days I drop more stitches than I complete. These scarves?" She gestured at the rainbow monstrosity in her lap. "I know they're ugly as hell. They're also proof I showed up today and made something, anyway."

She picked up the needles again. The clicking resumed, uneven and defiant.

Diane said, "There's just today. And what you choose to do with it."

I stared at her hands, shaking and fumbling, but still moving.

Gerald said, "You played Carnegie Hall?"

"In another life."

Linda said, "Do you miss it?"

"Every day." She didn't look up from her knitting. "But missing it doesn't bring it back. So, I make scarves and show up here."

"Someone told me it gets easier," Diane said. "She was lying. But I'll keep hoping."

Michelle leaned forward. "How? How can you hold on to hope?"

Diane's needles kept clicking. “Losing hope costs more than going home to an empty apartment and a violin I can't play anymore. Here, I don't have to perform hope.”

Martin surprised me when he said, “Not pretending gives me a chance to breathe. That's enough to keep me coming back.”

Rebecca said, “Some days that's all I bring here. Just the hope that next week might be different.”

“Beats the alternative,” Robert said. “Giving up, I mean. Not the sex.”

CHAPTER 26

Tuesday, July 14

The Corner Cafe smelled like bacon grease and pumpkin pie—the kind of smell that convinced you everything was going to be fine, even when the evidence suggested otherwise.

A woman in a yellow uniform led us to a booth by the window without asking if we had a preference. The vinyl squeaked as we settled in. The laminate tabletop had a repair strip across one corner that had begun to peel.

The menus were laminated and had photographs of food made to look fit for the gods. I opened mine and studied it with more attention than it deserved.

"The eggs are reliable," Rebecca said, without looking up. "The pancakes are ambitious. And their coffee is a crime against humanity."

"I'll have the coffee."

"Of course, we will." She smiled. "This was a great idea. But I'm not sure I picked the best place to eat."

From somewhere behind the pass-through window, something metal hit something metal and a radio was playing music.

The woman in yellow returned. Rebecca ordered coffee, eggs, and wheat toast. I ordered eggs, coffee, and a side of bacon that I probably wouldn't finish.

A white coffee cup arrived first — as heavy as a mug. I wrapped both hands around it. The ceramic was thick — the kind designed to survive dishwashers, careless handling, and the indifference of customers.

I turned it in my hands. "Perfect."

Rebecca said, "The coffee?"

"The cup."

"What? … Oh, yes. I like it too. Nice and heavy."

I said, "It helps."

"Sure does."

I took a sip. "It tastes like someone read about coffee once and decided to have a go."

Rebecca considered her cup. "It tastes like a decision made in haste and never revisited."

"It tastes like my first marriage would have tasted," I said, "if I'd had one."

Rebecca smiled. "My marriage tastes exactly like this. And I still drink it every morning."

"Is that love or stubbornness?"

"With Steve?" She tilted her head. "Genuinely hard to tell...But seriously. Yeah. He's the love of my life."

Outside the window, a dog tied to a parking sign was watching pigeons with profound interest.

"That dog," Rebecca said. "He's not going to do anything about the birds."

"No," I said. "But the commitment is admirable."

"There's something to be said," Rebecca said, "for knowing your limitations and watching pigeons, anyway."

The radio behind the pass-through shifted to a love song. The melody was present, but the feeling was missing. It reminded me of a word you know but can't quite place.

"Steve showed up at my door at midnight," Rebecca said, "the first week we were dating. I'd mentioned offhand that I'd never seen the original Rocky. He had the DVD and a bag of microwave popcorn, and this expression like he was delivering urgent medical supplies."

"Was the popcorn good?"

"The popcorn was terrible. How can a man burn popcorn in a microwave?" She laughed. "And it was cold."

"Cold popcorn. The stuff of holidays."

"Sadly, it wasn't Christmas. Steve got distracted on the drive over."

"By what?"

"He says traffic," she looked at her coffee. "I think he was nervous."

"Did you tell him it was terrible?"

"I told him it was the best popcorn I'd ever had."

"And?"

"Thirty years later, he still burns the popcorn every time we watch a movie." She paused. "I've never told him."

I thought about Paul and the Danish from the bakery on Wolf Boulevard. How he drove past two closer bakeries to get to that one. How he'd learned which ones I liked before I'd thought to tell him.

"Paul irons his socks," I said.

Rebecca looked up.

"Not the bottoms. Just the top. He says it keeps the elastic from degrading."

"Does it?"

"I've never looked it up. I'm afraid he might be right."

The unguarded laugh arrived before she could make it smaller.

The eggs came. The woman in yellow set them down with the efficiency of someone who had done this a thousand times and expected a just reward. She refilled our coffee without being asked, which we both accepted as the gift it was.

At a nearby table, a family was finishing breakfast: two parents, two children. The younger one — maybe four — had constructed a small landscape out of toast crusts and jelly packets. The older one was ignoring this with the elaborate disinterest of a sibling who had decided to be above such things.

The mother reached across and moved the jelly packets away, without breaking her conversation. The child relocated them without looking up. Neither parent acknowledged that it happened.

"My daughter used to arrange her peas," Rebecca said. "She didn't eat them. She just liked to sort them by size."

"She didn't like them?"

"She became a vegetarian at fourteen." Rebecca cut her toast into quarters. "I choose to interpret that as a win."

"Bold reframe."

"Reframing is a practiced skill." She looked at her eggs. "For survival."

The family's younger child was reaching for another jelly packet. The older one, without looking up from his own plate, slid one across the table. The gesture was so practiced it seemed unconscious.

"What did you do?" Rebecca asked. "Before teaching."

"I was going to ask you the same thing."

"I've always been a pharmacist at heart," she said. "When I was nineteen, I got a job at a drugstore." She looked at her hands briefly, then away.

"I loved teaching."

"What did you love about it?"

"I loved the moment when a kid who thought they hated reading found a book that didn't feel like reading," I said. "Something changes in their faces when it happens." I turned my mug in my hands. "You can't manufacture it. The magic of learning to love literature either happens or it doesn't."

Rebecca was quiet for a moment, letting it be what it was. "I love when a patient finally understands their medication," she said. "Not just the instructions on the bottle. What it's doing inside them."

She looked at her coffee. "People are less frightened of things they understand." She put food on her fork. "Other medications people trust when they should be running from them."

Chewing, she considered before adding, "I think sometimes understanding just gives you better ways of coping with fear."

Outside, a woman was yelling at the dog. She had the intensity of someone who believed she was right. The dog's eyes told a different story.

"She knows she's going to lose to the dog," Rebecca said.

"Then why keep arguing?"

"Maybe she thinks stopping feels like giving in." Rebecca picked up her coffee.

"Strange thing to do. Yell at a dog who is just doing what he was made to do."

The woman outside used a napkin to clean up the dog's waste, put it into a little bag, and came back into the diner.

"The eggs were good," I said.

"Told you."

When the check came, Rebecca reached for it.

"You don't have to," I said.

"I invited you." She left a tip more generous than the waitress deserved.

"Do you think you'll come next week?" Rebecca asked.

"Yes," I said.

We slid out of the booth. The vinyl squeaked again, the same note as before.

CHAPTER 27
Tuesday, July 14

A delivery truck idled at the curb, its hazards blinking in a rhythm that almost matched the song still half-playing in my head — the one from the radio, the one I still couldn't name.

"I'm not ready to go home," Rebecca said.

"Neither am I."

We started walking. We went past a gift store, the abandoned dry cleaner, and a bookstore with a hand-lettered sign in the window that said USED, LOVED, AVAILABLE. This seemed like a personal ad as much as anything else.

"I used to read a book a week," she said. "Before."

"I read slower now," I said.

"I reread the same paragraph," Rebecca said. "Four, five times. Then I put the book down and tell myself I'll finish it later."

"Do you?"

"No," she started walking again. "I have fourteen bookmarks in fourteen books. Steve says I have optimism."

"What do you call it?"

She thought about this seriously. "Evidence," she said. "That I still intend to."

We walked half a block in comfortable silence.

A child on a bicycle rode past. A woman on a stoop was drinking coffee and reading her phone.

"I was going to write a novel," I said.

Rebecca didn't react immediately. She kept walking.

"I had forty pages," I said. "Years of writing in the evenings." I watched the pavement in front of me. "I was finally getting somewhere with it."

"What happened to the forty pages?"

"They're on my laptop." I stepped around a crack in the sidewalk. "I haven't opened the file in eight months."

"You should. Read it and see."

"It's probably terrible," I said. "Most first novels are." I paused. "That's what I tell myself."

"Is that what you believe?"

She asked without pressure or the kindness that makes you feel managed. It was simply a question, offered plainly.

I stopped walking. "No," I said.

Rebecca nodded once.

We kept walking.

After a moment, she said, "I had a journal. I've been keeping one since I was thirty-two." She looked at a point somewhere ahead of us. "I haven't written in it since last year."

"What stopped you?"

"I couldn't read my own handwriting," she said. "I sat down to write and looked at the page from the week before, and I couldn't — I knew what the words said. I just couldn't make them out."

"That sucks."

"I told Steve the journal was full," she said. "He offered to buy me a new one."

"Did you let him?"

"It's on my nightstand." Her voice was perfectly level. "Still in the packaging."

A woman passed us walking a dog that appeared to be walking her. She was smiling about it, which seemed like the right response.

We reached the corner. The light was red.

The light changed. We crossed.

We were back in front of the diner. We'd walked a full circle without meaning to.

The woman in yellow was visible through the window, resetting a table.

"I'm not comfortable with our arrangement. The one with Paul."

She said, "What kind of arrangement?"

"The one where I'm fine," I said. "And he's worried but managing. And we both pretend the ratio is sustainable."

"Steve checks on me," she said. "I can tell because he texts me immediately after."

She watched the woman inside straighten a chair.

"Paul has even tied my shoes, with double knots," I said. "He doesn't ask. But he doesn't comment about why he needs to, either." I brushed hair off my face. "He started doing more for me, about six months ago."

We stood there, silent for a moment.

Rebecca said, "Managing is the right word for it."

The café's window reflected two women on a sidewalk, neither of them going home yet.

She said, "I'm thinking about retiring. Well, Steve thinks I should. I might."

I nodded.

"The forty pages," Rebecca said. "What is it about?"

I watched our reflections in the window.

"Someone losing something she didn't know she needed," I said. "Until it was gone. I thought I was writing about grief, after my mother died." I paused. "I don't think that's what it is anymore."

"What is it?"

"I don't know. That might be why I haven't opened it."

"The most frightening stories," Rebecca said, "are the ones you're still inside." She paused. "The only way to find out how they end is to keep reading."

"Same time next week," I said. It wasn't a question this time.

We walked to our cars. I didn't look back at the cafe, but I thought about the white mugs.

CHAPTER 28

Tuesday, July 14

The house was quiet. It was a different quiet than when Paul was simply in another room. The house had more square footage...more air.

I put my keys on the table and stood at the kitchen window, looking at the backyard going dark.

My phone rang while I was still standing there.

"Hey," I said.

Paul said, "Hey. How was the support group?"

"Good. Rebecca and I went to a cafe afterward."

"That's good."

I could hear the hotel room around him — the silence of anonymous space, the hum of climate control.

"How are you doing?" he asked. "Really."

"I'm fine," I said.

"Joy."

"I mean it. I'm good."

He said, "You sound off."

"I sound like someone who is okay."

"I just wanted to check in. I've been thinking about you. I've been thinking about whether I should come home early."

"Don't."

He said, "I'm just saying I could."

"I don't need you to come home and check on me."

"That's not what I said."

"It's what you meant."

The silence had a different texture now.

"I worry about you," he said. "That's not something I'm going to apologize for."

"I know you worry."

"Then what?"

"The ratio, Paul." The words arrived before I had finished deciding to say them. "The arrangement where I'm fine and you're worried but managing...managing me, and we both pretend that's sustainable." I could hear the edge in my voice. "That's what we have. That's what we've built."

He was quiet.

He said, "I like helping you."

"You track my medication and you adjust your schedule without telling me." My voice had steadied into something I didn't entirely recognize. "And I have let all of it happen. I have accommodated all of it and called it *love.* But I am so tired."

The silence on his end was the kind that meant the words had landed and he was inside them.

"I'm trying to take care of you," he said.

"I know."

"Then I don't understand what you're upset about."

"I know you're taking care of me. Sometimes I need help. But I'm tired of being taken care of. Sometimes, care has a shape, and the shape doesn't leave room."

"Room for what."

"For me to be the one who knows what I need."

Another silence.

"You fell," he said. "Three times this year. The gym's parking lot. The kitchen. The hallway in March that you didn't tell me about until I noticed the bruise. You forgot your medication. You don't eat the way you should."

"I know you love me."

"Then tell me what I'm doing wrong. Tell me how to be the person who doesn't worry about you."

I didn't say anything.

"Because the alternative," he said, "is watching you get worse and doing nothing. And I can't."

I heard him take a deep breath. "I can't do that."

I stood at the kitchen window with the phone against my ear.

"I saw you crying in the driveway," I said. "Before you left. I was at the window.

He didn't answer right away. When he did, his voice had the quality of loss. "I know. I saw you as I pulled out."

He said, "I'm not going to pretend I'm fine. I'm not fine. I'm frightened every day. There is stuff going on that I need to talk to you about. Not now. Not over the phone."

"About me?"

“We’ll talk when I come home.”

“You don’t need to come home early.”

“I'm not going to stop worrying,” he said. “You can be angry with me for it. That's fair. But I'm not going to stop caring.”

“I know,” I said. “That's not what I want.”

“Then what do you want?”

“I don't know,” I said. “I think I wanted you to know I'm tired.” I paused. “I'm sorry.”

“Don't be,” he said.

“I should let you sleep,” I said. “Good night, Paul.”

“Good night.”

I put the phone down on the counter and stood there for a moment. The house had the same square footage of quiet it had had an hour ago. It felt different now. More inhabited, somehow, though nothing had changed.

CHAPTER 29

Wednesday, July 15

Paul never called.

CHAPTER 30

Thursday, July 16

It started in the morning with a reasonable errand. The store parking lot was half-empty. A plastic bag moved in the wind — lifting and dropping, going nowhere. I sat in the car and watched it.

When I recognized what I was doing, I also recognized that this was a displacement, a substitute for something I was avoiding.

Avoidance had grown so familiar that I could observe it with something close to admiration. It seemed a shame that there was no certification for it.

I went inside. Three notebooks seemed more than I would need. I got them, anyway. I also bought pens, ones with black gel and fine tips.

In the produce aisle, I found a pre-packaged salad and tossed it into my basket.

I stood in the snack aisle longer than made sense and chose chips, a soda I hadn't had since my twenties, and a chocolate bar I put back and then retrieved. These were the small negotiations of a person who was not taking care of herself but knew that she should.

Blast it all, I want chocolate.

At the register, the cashier looked at my basket with the open curiosity of someone young enough to find other people's choices interesting.

CHAPTER 31

Thursday, July 16

I had told Rebecca, on the sidewalk outside the cafe, that I hadn't opened the file in months. I could still see the cafe window behind her, the two of us reflected in it slightly darker than we were. She had gone quiet when I said, "It's about someone losing something she didn't know she needed."

I opened the file and read the first page, then the second, then got up and made coffee, and came back and read from the beginning again.

The forty pages were better than I remembered. Not finished-good. It was rough in the wrong places, and one chapter lost its nerve halfway through. I used a metaphor that needed pulling back. But underneath, something moved.

The character had weight. She noticed the world with a precision that surprised me — not because I didn't recognize it, but because I did, the way you recognize your own handwriting in a letter you don't remember writing. For a moment it felt like being watched by yourself.

Her name was Eleanor. I had chosen her name with intention. It was the kind of name that didn't allow shortcuts. She lived in a river town, and the river was the thing the novel moved around without arriving at, the way you circle the thing you mean. The river first appeared on page seventeen. When it did, Eleanor stood on a bridge and looked down at water that moved so slowly it appeared still.

I had written: "She had the feeling, not for the first time, that stillness was just motion she hadn't learned to read."

I read that sentence three times. I had no memory of having written it. It sounded like someone who had understood, eight months before, something I was only now catching up to.

I was writing notes onto cards and pinning them on the wall. Eleanor's river. The town upstream. The words *second self* with a question mark. I gave Eleanor's life the quality of attention that becomes, at a certain point, indistinguishable from surveillance.

I stepped back and looked at my work. The cards covered most of the wall, some for Eleanor and some not yet categorized. The line between her story and the questions I had been carrying since Tuesday wasn't clear.

I wrote that Eleanor was standing at her kitchen sink, running the tap, watching the water move over her hands — hands that had started doing things she hadn't asked them to do. She noticed. Then she noticed the noticing. A second Eleanor took up residence behind the first, cataloguing everything with the patience of someone assigned a job they hadn't chosen.

I wrote until my right hand mistyped a word, stopped, and tried again. The second attempt was right.

Outside the kitchen window the light had turned the color of weak tea — that low, sideways light of late afternoon that arrives without announcement and changes the quality of everything while you're looking elsewhere. My coffee was cold. The chocolate bar sat in its wrapper beside the keyboard. The chips were gone. I opened the salad, took one bite, and tossed it into the garbage.

I checked the time. 6:47.

The first notebook was almost full. The index cards on the wall caught the light and threw small shadows, the thumbtacks leaving dark circles on the white paper. From where I sat, it looked less like research and more like something from a film about a person who had stopped sleeping.

I thought of Sarah sitting in the plastic chair beside Tom's wheelchair. She had described the moment she understood that loving someone and caring for someone was not the same work — that they pulled in different directions and that she was worn out by the distance between them.

Sarah said it the way you say a thing you have carried alone for a long time. She said in a room where no one was surprised by its weight.

Eleanor was still standing by the sink. A character couldn't spend a whole chapter in one place with her thoughts turning inward while the world held still. *Someone needs to arrive, leave, or speak.*

I wrote three sentences and deleted them, wrote two more, and one of them was right. I was trying to find what came after it when my phone rang.

CHAPTER 32

Thursday, July 16

Paul's name glowed on the screen. I looked at his name for a moment before I answered. It was 8:22...he was late in calling, but at least he called. Something in my chest was released, and the release made me aware — only in the letting go — that it had been held.

"Hey," I said.

"Hey." His voice came through thin with distance and fatigue. "Sorry. Long day."

"That's okay."

"How are you?" Paul's voice arrived through the phone smaller than his voice in a room, the way voices arrived smaller across distance.

I looked at the wall, the index cards in their uneven rows, Eleanor's river and my questions with the line between them dissolving in the low light.

"I opened the novel," I said.

"The forty pages," he said.

"Yes."

"And?"

"Better than I remembered." I turned away from the wall. "Which is a strange thing to find out about yourself."

I looked at the notebook, the pages dense with my handwriting, the letters larger than they used to be, taking up more space than they needed. "It doesn't sound like me. I don't remember being that person."

"Maybe you still are," he said.

Outside the window, the light was almost gone. I thought about Eleanor on her bridge, the water beneath her that looked still and wasn't.

"How are you?" I asked. "You sound tired."

"I am." He said it without the faint upward lift he sometimes used to signal that tiredness was manageable. "The project's been long."

I said, "Are you eating?"

He replied, "That's my line. I'm asking you."

"I'm eating...Badly, but I'm eating."

Paul said, "Yeah. Me too."

I said, "Are you alright?"

The pause had a different texture this time — the kind where someone is deciding how much of the truth to offer.

"I don't know," he said. "I keep thinking I called you last night. I remember picking up the phone. I went to sleep certain I'd done it."

Is this his excuse?

"But this morning I couldn't recall what you said. I hadn't called, had I? I don't show the call on my phone."

It wasn't a question.

He sounds concerned. Maybe he really thought he had called.

"No," I said.

"I was sure," he said. "That's the part that bothers me. Not that I forgot — that, I was sure."

"How long has this been going on? The memory." I asked.

"I don't know. A while." He let out a breath. "I thought it was just tiredness."

"Maybe it is," I said. "But you should see someone."

"I'll be back a week from Monday."

"Alright"

The index cards had lost their shadows, and the thumbtack circles had disappeared into the white. The whole arrangement looked, from where I sat, like nothing but paper.

Eleanor was still on the screen, the chapter unfinished, the one right sentence holding the place of what came next.

"Tell me about it," Paul said. "The novel. Tell me what's happening in it."

So, I told him about Eleanor, the river, and the water that moved so slowly it looked still. "Eleanor's hands do things she hasn't asked them to do.

Paul listened without interrupting, without offering solutions, present on the other end of the line — while the chapter assembled itself in the telling. Somewhere in the middle of describing Eleanor's hands, I stopped being certain whose hands I meant.

I kept going because Paul was there, and the screen was open, and the darkness outside was complete.

"She sounds real," he said when I stopped.

"She frightens me a little."

"Why?"

"Because she already knows things I'm still working out," I said. "She knew them down before I caught up to what I had written."

Paul was quiet.

I wrote the idea on the inside cover of the second notebook in handwriting that was still, on most days, legible.

Catching up to myself.

"Get some sleep," I said.

"You too."

After he hung up, the phone sat on the table beside the keyboard. The house settled into its sounds — the refrigerator, a car on the street, the silence of rooms where no one else was. I reached for the chocolate bar, opened it, broke off a piece, and looked at the screen.

Eleanor was still by the sink. Her hands were still under the water.

I moved her forward.

CHAPTER 33

Friday, July 17

The fiction awoke before I did. Eleanor was already standing when I opened the laptop. She was waiting with the patience of someone who had not been asleep at all but simply waiting there in the dark, holding the place of the next sentence until I was ready to write it.

I wasn't sure I was ready.

My morning had started ordinarily enough. Coffee, the pill, the brief negotiation with my body on the way to the kitchen that had become so habitual I barely registered it anymore — either adaptation or surrender, and I had stopped trying to determine which.

I put my fingers on the keyboard, and Eleanor responded.

It went well at first; the way writing goes well when something has been loosened the night before. The words arrived in the right order. Eleanor watched me write her; with the expression I had been trying to find for her since the beginning of the novel.

I wrote for an hour without stopping.

Eleanor moved through her morning as if the gravity of grief had thickened overnight. Her arms lagged, despite her intentions. The floor felt colder than it should have. She made the small negotiations and adjustments that accumulated into a day.

She made toast and burned it. The smell turned sharp and bitter, but she ate it anyway, chewing through the charcoal edge. Crumbs scattered across the counter and clung to her wrists.

She stood at the window and watched a neighbor she had never spoken to walking a dog. The leash clicked softly against the metal tag. The dog paused to nose at a patch of grass.

Eleanor felt a small, unreasonable pang. Twenty feet of pavement separated them. Twenty feet between her front door and the world, and all the conversations she had not had.

My day disappeared into Eleanor's world, until Paul called and broke the spell. When darkness came, I reluctantly went to bed.

CHAPTER 34

Saturday, July 18

I awoke ready to return to Eleanor's world. Eleanor's life on the page, and the sentences forming around her that I hadn't planned to write, had apparently been waiting with the same patience Eleanor had. So quietly, so incrementally, that no one in her world had noticed. Possibly including Eleanor herself.

Eleanor was at her kitchen table, looking at what I had written, recognizing it the way you recognize something you have known for a long time without having the words for it.

The words are always the last thing to arrive. Everything else — the body, the behavior, the years of small departures — was already there, waiting for the language to catch up.

My coffee went cold. My stomach rumbled. *When did I last eat? Yesterday? No.* I drank what remained of the cold coffee and kept writing.

She had not waited for time to take things from her. She had begun the work herself, quietly and without ceremony, leaving rooms before she was asked to go, as if departure chosen was less terrible than departure forced — not understanding yet that the room doesn't know the difference, and neither, in the end, does the person who has left it.

I stopped. I read the last sentence again. Outside the window, the flat white sky had deepened, the way it deepened when the morning was deciding whether to become something. A car moved down the street. Somewhere nearby, a door closed.

I looked at the words. My hands were on the keyboard, and the tremor was doing what the tremor did. I understood — not gradually, not reluctantly, but all at once, the way you understand things you have been carefully not understanding for a very long time.

The words are coming faster. Too fast.

Not faster than I could think them — faster than my hands could manage. My fingers mistyped the words and lost the thread while my fingers were still moving. I did what I had set up months ago and never used: switched to dictation, clicked the microphone, and began to speak.

I spoke of every room she had left, the conversations she had shortened, the music she had stopped playing before time could make stopping necessary — because possible and imperfect were worse, somehow, than impossible and clean. She had been so afraid of being diminished in the eyes of the people she loved that she had diminished herself first, with the efficiency of someone who had decided the outcome and was simply managing the timeline.

I stopped, took a sip of the cold coffee, and spoke again.

The cruelest part, Eleanor thought, *was that she had called it strength. Had believed she was protecting the people she loved from the spectacle of aging. She had not understood until this morning, that protection offered from behind a closed door was not protection at all.*

I heard my own voice say the words and kept going.

She had been so busy managing her exit that she had forgotten she was still here. Still in the room. Still capable of wanting things. She could feel it now — the wanting, which she had packed away so carefully that she had almost convinced herself it was gone. It wasn't gone.

It had been waiting, the way the novel had been waiting in my closed computer.

Everything she had set down was still exactly where she had left it.

I stopped dictating.

The kitchen was very quiet.

Is my life waiting to be picked back up?

I sat with my hands on the table and the story of Eleanor on the screen. I could not say how long I sat there before my phone rang.

"Hey," I said.

"Hey." He sounded better than the night before, more present, though the fatigue was still there underneath. "How's the writing?"

How do I tell you?

"Eleanor is moving," I said. "She's been at it all morning."

"Good moving or complicated moving?"

I looked at the screen.

"She wrote something," I said. "That I didn't know she was going to write."

"What did she write?"

I read one sentence to him.

When I stopped reading, there was silence on the line. The space stretched and I reread the sentence, silently to myself. *She had been so busy managing her exit that she had forgotten she was still here.*

"Joy," he said.

Not a question. Not the careful version of my name he used when he was managing me. Just my name, the way he used to say it, before we both learned to be so careful with each other.

He said, "Is it Eleanor, or you?"

"I don't know yet," I said. "Both."

He was quiet for a long moment, giving the question the room it needed.

"I've missed you," he said. "I didn't know how to say that without it sounding like an accusation."

"I've missed you too," I said.

The phone held us for a moment.

"I'll be home in about a week." he said. "We'll talk."

"Love you."

After he hung up the phone, I reached for the chocolate bar and broke off another piece.

I turned the microphone back on.

CHAPTER 35

Saturday, July 18

I was still dictating when it started. I had time to think, *not now. The writing is flowing.* And then I had no thoughts about the story at all. It was replaced by my body refusing to move.

The chair. Stay on the chair.

The microphone was still open on my laptop. Eleanor's last words, "*I was broken,*" hung where I had just dictated them.

When did I take a pill?

My body asserted the one thing it had never stopped asserting — that it was here, it was real, and nothing occurring in this kitchen could happen outside its terms. I didn't reach for my phone. I couldn't move.

I forgot to take the pill.

A tightening had begun beneath my skin, beneath the muscle — somewhere I couldn't point to. My fingers drew in toward the palm, the way a hand closes in sleep. Except I was not asleep. I was watching it happen — watching from slightly too far away, the way you might watch something happening across a street before you understand it is happening to you.

I told my fingers to stop.

They didn't stop.

I told them again.

They drew the rest of the way in, slowly, with the unhurried finality of something decided elsewhere, and the tightness moved up through the wrist and into the forearm, and my shoulder pulled inward. My whole right side reorganized itself around an instruction I hadn't given.

Then the stillness came.

I need a pill.

I formed the intention to stand. Sent it.

It went nowhere. Not blocked. Not refused. The line between what I meant and what happened disappeared, the way a room goes silent when someone stops speaking and the silence has time to settle. I tried to shift my weight...the way a physical therapist had taught me. Rock slightly; let the movement find the side door. I assembled the instructions and sent them.

They never arrived.

One.

The wooden edge of the chair pressed into the back of my thigh. The grain of it through my jeans, the exact pressure of it, the way it would leave a mark.

Two.

My pulse in my curled fingers. Small. Continuous. My body conducted its own business.

Three.

I sent the instructions again.

Four.

Nothing.

My breath was shallow. I could hear it now, like I'd never heard it before; and had never had a reason to. That small sound, in and out, and underneath it I heard the refrigerator, and outside a dog barking...these ordinary sounds arranged around me like furniture in a room I could see and not move through.

My eyes went to the window.

I could do that.

The thin light moved through clouds, touched the street, and lifted away. My eyes moved to find it and went slightly past, overshooting, catching on the empty bird feeder before coming back. A small wrong tracking, there and gone. The neighbor's hedge. A strip of pale sky. Visible. Continuing. And below all of that, a body sitting in a chair that had stopped taking requests, pulse in the fingers, breath in the chest, and nothing else available.

The dog barked again.

I tried to lift my right foot. The toe strained — a small involuntary hitch, a trying — and then nothing.

I didn't know how long I had been sitting there.

I tried again to shift my weight, sending the instructions carefully, the way you'd lower your voice to get a child's attention.

Nothing.

The word, *broken*, surfaced somewhere below language and sank before I could fully reach the thought.

Timing, I thought. The word landed flat. Like a joke told in an empty room.

I reached for humor. But I couldn't find it.

The piano.

The weight of its keys. The action of them. The piano returned pressure in exact proportion to what you gave it.

The classroom.

The last day when the door closed behind me. *I'd chosen to leave. I always leave.*

Afraid.

The thought stayed with me...the word didn't step back. I sat there, suspended in time.

My fingers uncurled.

Not because I asked, but because my body decided to release, moving in its own time, indifferent to what had just arrived in me, indifferent to what was still arriving. One finger, then another. The last one, slow, considering whether it was ready to open.

I looked at my open hand.

Broken was the word under all the other words. The word I had been arranging my life around. It sat in the kitchen with me now, plain and without ceremony. The chair was solid beneath me. *I'm afraid* — the realization became clear, emerging from deep within me, settling as truth in the same way the chair was under me. Tangible. Present. Unarguable. Mine.

CHAPTER 36

Saturday, July 18

I tried again to shift my weight. The intention formed. A beat passed before my body followed. Time passed without reliable measurement. My body was still recalibrating...cognition was still catching up.

Then I folded. It was not exactly a decision. My body made a choice that my mind didn't initiate. Not falling, more like a sliding downward done in slow motion. My legs found the floor, paused before lowering the rest of my body. My left hand steadied me against the cabinet as I went down.

My side felt the slight unevenness of the landing register. I had a moment — *Yes. The floor is there.* — and then my back found the cabinet and the whole of me settled against it, inward and downward, until I was on the floor. The linoleum was cool through my jeans. Cooler than expected. I pressed the back of my head lightly against the cabinet. Solid.

I left myself behind. I chose to leave.

CHAPTER 37
Saturday, July 18

Getting up from the floor took longer than it should have. Not from the episode — that had passed, with the circuitry restored to the baseline my brain maintained. Only heaviness remained...I felt exhausted.

I reached for the edge of the drawer and pushed...with more attention than the motion required...initiating each stage with the deliberateness of someone who had learned not to assume. My weight shifted forward. My feet found the floor and held there a beat before committing.

I stood for a moment, just stood, my hand still on the cabinet, just in case.

The laptop was on the table, the red light still steady, the microphone still open. The story of Eleanor was on the screen, the cursor blinking. I reached over and turned off the microphone. The dictation light went out. I opened the pill bottle and took one.

I walked to the cupboard. Paul's blue mug was where I had put it, beside my white one, both pushed to the back. I took them out, both hands shaking from the effort. Set them on the counter side by side. I stood there looking at them, then left them where they were and walked out of the kitchen.

Then I went into Paul's office and stopped in front of the bookshelf.

The photograph from Vermont.

It had been a hiking weekend, one of Paul's ideas that I had agreed to, having the vague suspicion that it would involve more physical effort than I was prepared for, which it did. There was a trail that ended at a small overlook above a valley. The trees below were in full color. The air was sharp and cold and clean.

A stranger, another hiker, offered to take our photograph. In it, Paul was laughing at something I had just said. I didn't remember what I had said. I remembered the quality of his laugh — unguarded.

I set the photograph down and looked at my hands. The tremor was at its usual amplitude now; the post-episode increase was gone.

I wrote sentences in my head. This part did not need to be recorded. It did not belong to Eleanor.

She had not waited to be diminished. She had begun the work herself — quietly, without ceremony — stepping out of life before anyone thought to ask her to leave.

I picked up the photograph again and carried it to the couch and sat down with it in my lap. Outside, two birds crossed each other's calls.

CHAPTER 38

Saturday, July 18

I heard his key in the lock before I heard his car in the driveway. I had been sitting on the couch with the Vermont photograph in my hands for longer than I knew.

He is more than a week early. We just spoke…when was it? Today. Though it felt like days had passed.

The key turning. The sound of the door opening, which I had heard a thousand times and had not, until this moment, understood I had been cataloguing.

"Joy?"

His voice from the entryway, the same voice that had come through the phone thin with distance and fatigue, now full, present, and here.

"In here, Paul," I said.

His footsteps crossed the entryway. The rhythm of his walking had a slight hesitation I had been noticing for months without naming it — I heard it now, three steps and then the fourth arriving a beat late, and I held the knowledge of it the way I had been holding the photograph.

He appeared in the doorway. His work shirt was rumpled. He took in the room the way he took in most things — quietly, without announcing what he was doing.

He looked at me.

I looked back.

Something moved across his face that I didn't have a name for — not relief exactly, not surprise, something more interior than either. More like the expression of a person who has been holding a breath they didn't know they were holding and has just let it go.

He set his bag down.

"You're early," I said.

"I wanted to be home." He came into the room and sat beside me on the couch, not at the careful distance he had often been maintaining for a year and a half, but close to me, the way he used to sit. He looked at the photograph in my hands. "Vermont."

I said, "Before the diagnosis. Before I changed...we changed."

He looked at it for a moment. His eyes moved to my face and then back to the photograph. I understood he was doing what I had been doing — looking at us, how we were before.

He was quiet.

Outside the window, the sky had gone the deep blue that wasn't quite dark, and the crickets had started; the sound of them coming through the glass steady and unhurried.

"How was your day?" he asked.

The question he always asked. The question I always answered in the managed way, presenting *fine*. I felt the habit of it rise and decided that I didn't have to pretend.

"Long," I said. "And strange." I looked at the photograph. "I think I've been gone for a while. And I think I'm starting to find my way back."

He didn't ask what I meant. He simply sat with it, probably turning it over or making room for it.

His hand found mine on the cushion between us. Just his hand on mine, the warmth of it, the weight. The tremor in my hand stilled, held at bay by his hand.

"I'm sorry," I said.

He kissed my forehead and asked, "For what?"

"For being so far away."

"I've been far away too," he said.

"Are you alright?" I asked.

"I will be," he said. "There are things I need to tell you. Not tonight." He turned back to me. "But soon."

He squeezed my hand.

The south window held the last of the blue light. Almost dark now. The room was growing dim around us, but neither of us moved to turn on a lamp.

CHAPTER 39

Sunday, July 19

The story about Eleanor was open. I hadn't written anything new all morning. A sound came from the bathroom. The noise was measured, intermittent, and made me close my laptop.

The bathroom door was open. Paul was on one knee, his back to the door. He had a power drill in his right hand. Beside him was an assortment of tools and bathroom gadgets.

He was lining up a bracket against the tile, his left hand steadying while his right hand gripped the drill harder.

The drill bit went in. He moved the bracket a fraction, checked the level, and made another mark. His jaw was set the way it was when he was solving something that required his full attention.

He set the drill down, reached for the level, checked it against the wall, made a small sound in the back of his throat—satisfaction, the kind that belongs only to the person making the measurement.

I stood in the doorway and watched him work. My right hand was doing its thing against the doorframe. I pressed my thumb into my palm until it stilled.

He reached for the drill again. His right hand closed around the handle. A tremor was there...barely visible. He gripped the drill, and the tremor stilled, and he drove the first screw into the anchor, and the bracket held.

This isn't a tremor from stress.

He moved to the second anchor point. Measured. Marked. Drilled. He paused to brush his graying hair off his face.

Gerald had said that his body accepted aging before he had. He said his pride was still in transit.

Paul attached a grab bar, tested it with both hands, leaned his weight into it, pulled, and checked for any give. There was none. He tested it again, then once more.

He turned his attention to the showerhead. The old one was already off and a new bracket installed. His right hand was screwing on the new showerhead. He placed the handheld head into the bracket and tested the swivel.

Then he looked at what he'd done.

He picked up an instruction sheet, turned it over, compared a picture to the mounting hardware, and set it back down.

"Paul."

He turned. "Hey."

"When did you go to the hardware store?"

"This morning." He looked at the level. "While you were writing."

I looked at the fold-down bench waiting to be mounted. “Looks good.”

“I've been meaning to do it.”

“The bench,” I said. “Is that necessary?”

He looked at it. “It will be eventually.” He looked back at me. “I'd rather it be there before it’s needed.”

“The bench will work there,” I said, “against that wall.”

He looked at the wall, nodded once, already calculating.

I watched him: measure, drill, anchor, test. He tested it the same way he'd tested the grab bar: weight, pull, check for give.

He said, “There's something I wanted to tell you.”

He didn't look up from the drill case. “The scan,” he said. “Little Rock. I want to drive you.”

I was quiet.

“I know you were going to drive yourself.” He closed the drill case. Picked it up. “I know you didn't ask.” He finally looked at me. “I'm going to take the day off. I want to be there.”

“The DAT scan? Okay,” I said.

He picked up the drill case and the empty packaging. He carried everything past me into the hall.

From the kitchen came the sound of the drill case being set down. I stayed where I was, looking at the bathroom improvements. Then, I heard Paul washing his hands.

I put my hand on the grab bar nearest to the tub. I felt the solidity of the thing he had put on the wall. I was grateful, but not.

CHAPTER 40

Monday, July 20

Paul said, "Would you like to take a walk?"

This was unusual. Paul never took a walk. Plus, it was 7:30, which meant we should have been watching the local news while eating dinner.

"A walk?" I said, looking up from my laptop, where I'd been scrolling through videos of other people's lives.

The floor was still in my body somewhere — the cool of the linoleum, the pressure of the cabinet. I hadn't told Paul about the episode...or what I'd learned about myself.

I looked down at the end table, at my dinner wrapped in cellophane. Steam rose from the meatloaf, mashed potatoes, mixed vegetables, and a bite-sized, overcooked cake.

"Around the block. Fresh air. Exercise." He was already putting on his shoes.

I watched him lace up. "Are those shoes new?"

"Walking shoes."

I said, "It's almost dark."

He straightened, testing his weight on the cushioned soles. "That's what streetlights are for."

"We never walk around the block."

"Then we're overdue." He held out my sneakers like an offering. His eyes had the same wide, hopeful quality they'd had on our wedding day, as if he were asking me to trust him with something important. "Come on. The dishes can wait."

The dishes had been waiting since breakfast. And I really wasn't thrilled about the meatloaf.

I put on my shoes. Paul waited patiently by the door, keys in hand, even though we weren't going anywhere that required keys.

"Why do you have keys?"

"In case we decide to drive."

"We're walking around the block."

He jingled the keys. "You don't know. We might get ambitious. We could walk downtown. Then we'd need the car to get home."

"That's not how any of this works. The car would still be here. In the driveway. Someone would need to walk back to get it."

He frowned at the keys in his hand as if they might explain themselves. "Well, you never know when you'll need keys. Boy Scout motto."

"That's not the Boy Scout motto."

"It should be." He opened the door, caught his shoulder on the doorframe, adjusted, and gestured me through with a flourish. "After you."

The evening air hit us like a warm, damp towel in the face. We started down the driveway. Our shoes made satisfying crunching sounds on the gravel.

"So," he said as we reached the sidewalk. "How was your day?"

"Fine." I immediately felt off. *Why did I say fine?*

"Just fine? Nothing exciting? No celebrity sightings?"

I kicked at a loose stone. My foot didn't quite connect the way I'd intended. "I went to the grocery store."

"That's exciting."

"I bought milk."

"Thrilling." He grinned at me. "The crowds must have been wild."

"A woman was arguing with the cashier about expired coupons."

"God help that cashier."

"There was a binder."

Paul laughed. "A binder? Like, organized coupons?"

"Color-coded tabs. The cashier looked terrified."

"That's someone who takes grocery shopping seriously. We should aspire to that level of commitment."

I bumped his shoulder with mine. "We can barely commit to doing the dishes."

"That's different. Dishes don't have expiration dates." He paused. The cicadas were starting up in the trees, providing the summer evening with a pulse. "Besides, tomorrow someone will definitely handle it."

"Tomorrow, someone *probably* will."

We turned the corner. A man was watering his lawn. He waved at us. Water arced from the hose as his arm moved. Paul waved back.

"How was your day?" I asked.

"Met with boring people about boring things." He thrust his right hand into his pocket. "Then I came home to eat boring frozen dinners in front of boring news."

"We lead such glamorous lives."

Paul laughed. "We're practically celebrities."

"Should we get sunglasses? For when the paparazzi show up?"

He said, "Definitely. And a yacht."

I touched his shoulder. "Where would we keep a yacht?"

"The bathtub. Obviously."

Silence settled between us for a few steps. A car passed. Its headlights swept across us.

Paul stopped walking and studied a tree in someone's yard with the intensity of an art critic. "Is that tree leaning?"

I looked. The oak stood straight, its bark rough and dark in the fading light. "No."

"It looks like it's leaning."

"It's straight."

He tilted his head. "That one branch is definitely going left."

"Branches do that."

Paul shook his head critically. "Rebellious branch. Refusing to conform."

We started walking again. My right foot caught on the concrete. The toe scraped instead of lifting. I heard the scuff, felt the slight drag—step, scuff, step, scuff. I focused on lifting my toes higher, on making my foot do what it was supposed to do.

"If I were a branch," Paul said, "I'd grow sideways too. Straight up is boring."

"You're a very silly man."

"Thank you."

A smell drifted over the fence from two houses down. Charcoal smoke and meat, sweet barbecue sauce caramelizing. It smelled like six summers ago, the last Fourth of July party we hosted. Paul had manned the grill with a beer in his hand, spatula in the other, conducting an orchestra of sizzling hot dogs and burgers.

My stomach growled loud enough that Paul heard it.

"Are you hungry?" he asked.

"Starving."

"We could walk back."

I shook my head. "The block isn't that big. I'll survive."

"It's bigger than you think. There are hidden depths to this block." He gestured dramatically at the sidewalk stretching ahead of us, his voice climbing half an octave. "Mystery. Wonder. That one house with the weird lawn gnome collection."

"That's four streets over."

"Four streets of adventure." He was smiling too widely, talking too fast—the way he did when he was trying to convince himself as much as me.

A dog barked at us from behind a fence. Its tail was wagging so hard that its whole back end wiggled. Its wet nose pressed against the chain-link. Paul stopped, planted his feet, and barked back. "WOOF!"

The sound came out loud enough that a porch light came on two houses down.

The dog's ears went flat. Its tail stopped mid-wag. It tilted its head, confusion replacing excitement, then backed away three steps.

"Did you just bark at a dog?" I asked.

"We were having a conversation."

"He can't understand your bark.."

He watched the confused retriever. "You don't know that. Maybe we had a very meaningful exchange."

"About what?"

"The futility of fences. The nature of freedom." He watched the dog circle nervously, clearly trying to figure out what had just happened. "Whether squirrels are worth chasing when your time might be limited."

The words hung between us. He meant it as a joke. His delivery had been light, but it still landed off-center.

He opened his mouth. Closed it. Shook his head.

"I think I hurt his feelings," Paul added quickly.

"You definitely confused him."

"Same thing."

We walked on. The sidewalk was uneven here, pushed up by tree roots into little peaks and valleys. I stepped over each crack with exaggerated care, focusing on lifting my feet properly.

"Remember when we first moved here?" he asked. "You said the neighborhood was 'charming.'"

"It is charming."

"You said 'charming' in that voice you use when something isn't charming at all."

I laughed. "I did not."

"You absolutely did. Same voice you use when my mother serves that casserole."

"Your mother's casserole is lovely."

He raised an eyebrow. "It has raisins in it. In a casserole. With chicken."

I caught my toe on a particularly large crack and stumbled slightly. Paul's hand shot out and caught my elbow. My fingers gripped his arm harder than necessary.

"And water chestnuts," I said, steadying myself. "Like someone designed it specifically to punish taste buds."

I let go of his elbow.

I said, "It was...interesting."

"That's the voice." He grinned at me, the streetlight catching his face, and for a moment, he looked exactly like he did ten years ago. "You're very polite when you hate things."

"I don't hate the neighborhood."

"Just the raisin casserole."

"Okay, the raisin casserole." I paused. "And maybe the wind chimes."

"Almost everyone here has wind chimes."

"Yes. I hate the wind chimes."

"See? Honesty. That's what I'm talking about." He took a breath, let it out slowly, and squared his shoulders. "We should be honest about more things."

"Like what?"

"Like..." He stopped walking and looked at me. His mouth opened, closed, and started again. "Like how you've been looking at me lately. Like you're memorizing things." His shoulders dropped.

I turned away, focusing on a house across the street—anywhere but his face. The night sounds seemed very loud suddenly. Crickets. A distant car. My own heartbeat.

"I'm not."

"The way I hold my fork. How I tie my shoes. What I look like when I'm not paying attention." His voice was gentle, but there was steel underneath. "You think I don't notice, but I do."

My right hand trembled at my side. I clenched it, hiding the movement.

"We should talk about it," he said. "Your diagnosis. Are you afraid you might start forgetting?"

I wanted to laugh but couldn't. *My memory is fine. Is Paul's? My body is betraying me, not my mind. Will that always be true?*

But I also wanted to tell him, *yes. I am memorizing you.*

"Not tonight," I said. The words came out sharper than I intended. "Please. Not tonight."

"Okay," he said. "Not tonight."

We started walking again, but everything felt different now—heavier, more real.

I said, "Bridge Street. We walked more than a block."

A jogger passed us going the opposite direction, hair swinging, earbuds in, moving at a pace that made me tired just watching. She left a wake of coconut sunscreen smell and determination.

"I used to jog," I said, watching her disappear around the corner.

"When?"

"College. I was very athletic."

Paul snorted. "You played intramural softball."

"Exactly. Athletic."

"You told me you were in right field because nobody hit it there."

"Strategy." I paused. "I was conserving energy for important things, like eating nachos in the dugout."

"You ate nachos during games?"

"Someone had to. It was a matter of team morale."

He laughed. "That's not team morale."

"The team's nachos weren't going to eat themselves. I was being selfless."

"That's not selfless."

"Besides, right field was perfect. You could see the whole field. The whole game. Everything at once."

We could see our house now, our porch light glowing yellow and warm. Moths circled it in dizzy loops, casting moving shadows. The blue recycling bin sat by the curb, forgotten since Friday morning.

"That's tomorrow's problem," Paul said, following my gaze.

"Let's say that about every problem."

"Agreed." He squeezed my hand.

The last of the fireflies were out, blinking, fighting against the darkening sky. One landed on my arm, its little feet tickling before it flew off. I tried to catch one in my cupped hands, missed, and tried again. My movements were slower than they used to be. My hands didn't quite close in time.

Paul joined me, reaching for the fireflies with exaggerated swoops.

"You're not going to catch one," I said.

"Watch me."

He didn't catch one, but he tried fourteen more times, each attempt more dramatic than the last, complete with sound effects and commentary. "This one's mine. I can feel it. No, wait, that's a moth."

I laughed. "Moths don't count."

"Moths should count."

"I'm saying moths don't count."

I was still laughing by the time we reached our driveway.

We stood there in the growing dark, the gravel crunching under our shoes as we shifted weight. The street was quiet now, except for the crickets and wind chimes making metallic music.

"That was nice," I said.

"Yeah." The lines around his eyes had deepened. His mouth was set in a way that said he was holding something back. "Joy, there's something I need to tell you."

"What?"

He opened his mouth, closed it, and shook his head.

"Tomorrow," he said finally. "I'll tell you tomorrow. Tonight, I just want to be with you."

"Paul, if something's wrong."

"It's nothing to worry about. I'm just not ready yet. Is that okay?"

I nodded, even though I wanted to push, because I understood not being ready. I'd not been ready for four years.

"We'll walk every night if you want," he said.

"Every night might be ambitious."

"Then twice a week. Wednesday and Saturday."

I touched his arm. "You love your schedules."

"I do love schedules." He took my right hand, holding it with both of his. "We'll add it to the calendar. Walk around the block with your wife. Bark at dogs. Fail to catch fireflies. Be together."

"That's a long calendar entry."

"Worth it."

We stood there, hands clasped, not moving.

He pulled me closer. "I'll hold you tight, even after tomorrow."

The word landed in my chest like a stone. *Tomorrow. Both a promise and a deadline.*

CHAPTER 41

Monday, July 20

Routine waited for us inside.

The house smelled like the vanilla candle I'd burned that morning and the faint mustiness of air conditioning that hadn't quite won against the humidity. The dishes were still in the sink, exactly where we'd left them.

"Want to watch something terrible on TV?" Paul asked.

"Always."

I ended up on the couch with ice cream eaten straight from the carton — cookies and cream for me, chocolate chip for him. Some cooking show was on...Paul muted the TV.

"The tree was definitely leaning," Paul said through a mouthful of ice cream.

"It absolutely was not."

"You just don't appreciate a good lean."

"There was no lean!"

"Tomorrow we're walking past it again, and I'm proving it."

"You're going to look like an idiot using a plumb line on a tree."

"Worth it." He took another bite. Some ice cream dripped onto his shirt. He looked down at it, then at me, and laughed. "Great. Now I match the dishes."

"We'll get you a bib."

Paul grinned. "And matching napkins. Very sexy."

"Very dignified."

"Add a bib to tomorrow's list of upgrades."

I tossed a pillow at Paul. He caught it and tucked it under his chin, laughing.

The cooking show ended. Another one started, then another.

At some point, Paul's breathing shifted into the slow rhythm of sleep, his head heavy on my shoulder.

I kept thinking about what Paul had said, about memorizing him.

I was also memorizing myself. The way my hand felt in moments when it was still. The way my feet moved without thinking down the sidewalk, heel and toe, heel and toe, not a single thought required. The simple freedom of driving a car — the automatic reach for the turn signal, the body knowing exactly what to do before the mind catches up. These things I had always done without noticing them. I was noticing them now.

I pulled out my phone, careful not to wake Paul, and typed.

Mom, something happened to me. And something is going on with Paul. Can we talk tomorrow?

I hit the send button.

The screen glowed in the dark room. Paul's breathing stayed steady beside me.

Recipient not found.

Mom would have known what to say. She would have known how to tell the difference between reasonable concern and the kind that eats you alive. She always did — that gift of hers, practical and clear-eyed, the way she could look straight at a hard thing and tell you what it was. I had wanted to give it to her: the true thing, named plainly, the way she had always taught me to name things. I had planned to tell her about my diagnosis. But when it came down to it, I couldn't bring myself to tell her. At the time, I decided *she has cancer; that's enough to deal with.*

Paul shifted in his sleep. His hand found my arm without waking up. I put the phone down.

I wish I had someone to talk to about the episode…about Parkinson's, and about Paul.

CHAPTER 42

Tuesday, July 21

I had my keys in my hand when Paul came out of the bedroom. He was dressed. Not in the clothes he wore around the house — in the clothes he wore when he was going somewhere: dark khakis and a beige shirt. He had his keys.

"I thought I'd come with you," he said.

I had decided to skip the support group meeting, so I could spend the day with Paul.

"To the grocery store?"

"Yes." He looked back at me with the expression he used when a decision had already been made, and he was presenting it as a suggestion out of courtesy.

"I can drive myself," I said.

He held the door open.

The morning was already warm, the wet warmth of a summer day that had decided early that it intended to be hot. I stood on the front step for a moment with my keys still in my hand and looked at Paul's car in the driveway.

Paul walked to his car and opened the passenger door. I understood that I was expected to sit in the passenger seat.

Since when does he open my door? Is he being old-fashioned? Romantic? …Or managing?

He closed my door, walked around, and got in. He adjusted the mirror, even though it didn't need adjusting, and backed down the driveway with both hands on the wheel.

I looked out the window at our street going past.

"Do you have the list?" Paul asked.

I handed it to him.

He read it at the next red light. Held it in his left hand and read it the way he read site plans — not once through but with the focused attention of a man organizing information into a sequence. Looking for inefficiencies. *He's probably planning a route through the store.*

"We can get the paper towels in the same aisle as the cleaning supplies," he said. "Save a trip."

I was right.

"I know where the paper towels are."

"Right." He set the list on the console between us.

The grocery store parking lot was fuller than I expected for Tuesday morning. But Paul found a space near the entrance.

He got out and came around to my side. I had already opened the door.

Maybe I should've waited.

We walked to the door, holding hands. Through the automatic doors, cool air chilled my arms. Paul took a cart from the row and steered it toward the produce section. I walked beside him.

It had been months since I had been here with Paul. He had always pushed the cart. I had always carried the list. He would disappear for ten minutes and come back with something that wasn't on the list but that he'd decided we needed.

Now he had the cart and the list.

He worked efficiently. Produce first: tomatoes, spinach, apples. He checked each item against the list and placed them in the cart with the same precision he brought to everything physical: the tomatoes away from the apples so nothing would bruise.

I reached past him to turn one of the tomato containers over to check the bottom, and he waited without comment.

In the bread aisle, he put the whole wheat in the cart, instead of our usual white bread. Then he looked at the list again.

"You have yogurt on here," he said. "The full-fat Greek or the low-fat?"

"Full-fat Greek is thicker."

"The low-fat might be healthier."

"I know what I want."

He put the full-fat yogurt in the cart.

Paul stopped in front of the frozen vegetables and compared two bags with concentration.

I drifted ahead toward the ice cream. I found the one I wanted without trying. It was the same ice cream I had been buying for years.

"That's a lot of sugar," Paul said. He was beside me now; the frozen vegetables were in the cart.

I looked at the container.

"And saturated fat." He wasn't unkind. He was reporting findings. "The dairy isn't great for inflammation either. There are some good alternatives."

"I know there are alternatives."

"Not in the regular dairy section. I saw a video. Said the soy-based ones have improved. It tastes almost like ice cream."

I stood with the ice cream container in my hands.

I thought about the evenings I had eaten it. The comfort of it — not the taste exactly, but the ritual. It was a small thing I still got to choose for myself, that asked nothing of my body, that existed entirely outside the system of management and optimization that illness had imposed on almost everything else I did. I realized Paul was now trying to manage my nutrition.

"You want to try an ice cream alternative?"

I put it back in the case. "I don't want ice cream. We had it last night."

Paul moved on to the next section, and I followed him. After Paul had gotten what he wanted from my list, we turned toward the checkout lanes.

I heard her before I saw her.

Carol's laugh always announced her presence before her arrival. Her laugh had made faculty meetings bearable for ten years. We used to sit together at a table in the Humanities Building, talking over lunch.

She was in the next aisle over, visible through the gap in the shelving. Her hair was shorter than I remembered. She hadn't seen us yet.

I should say something.

We came around the corner.

She looked up. "Joy."

I said, "Hi, Carol."

Her face did something complicated in the space of a second — surprise, then a brightness that arrived a beat late, then something that settled underneath the brightness and stayed there. "Joy," she said again as she walked toward us. "It's so good to — you look great."

"It's good to see you," I said. "How have you been?"

"Oh, you know." She gave the answer you gave when you didn't want to give an answer. Her eyes moved to Paul. And stayed.

"Paul." Her voice warmed. She stepped forward and touched his arm. "How are you holding up?"

"We're managing," Paul said. "It's been an adjustment."

"I can only imagine." She shook her head. "You're so good with her. I don't know how you do it."

"She does most of the work," Paul said.

"Still," Carol looked at me then — a quick look, the kind that checked a box without requiring engagement. Her eyes went back to Paul. "Is she getting out much? Getting some social time?"

I'm standing right here.

"Some."

Another brief glance at me, a smile directed somewhere in my vicinity. "And you're eating all right? I guess you're doing the cooking."

"We've been paying attention to that," Paul said, looking at the cart.

I thought about ice cream...and the list Paul carried and changed.

"I heard Dr. Patel is cutting back on her patient load," Carol said. "That must have been hard, losing that continuity."

What? No one told me.

"Yes. I got a letter about that. If Dr. Patel cuts Joy from her care, I'll find her a new neurologist," Paul said.

"Is she still writing?" Carol asked. "I always thought if anyone would find a way to keep busy, it'd be Joy."

"I'm writing a story."

Neither of them looked at me.

Carol was already saying something to Paul about the summer, about a conference she was presenting at in September, and then switched to telling him about a colleague who had taken early retirement. Paul listened, fully, with the slight forward tilt that meant he was tracking everything.

I looked toward the end of the aisle.

Carol's laugh came again — not the full one, a smaller version, responding to something Paul had said that I hadn't heard. She touched his arm again. She looked at me with the expression people used when they were looking at something that required them to be careful.

"You're so lucky to have him," she said to me. Directly. The first full sentence she had aimed at me in the entire conversation.

I looked at Paul and then at Carol.

"I know," I said.

Carol said goodbye to Paul. Then she looked at me and said it was so good to see me and that I looked wonderful and that I should take care of myself.

She turned and pushed her cart toward the checkout lanes.

Paul watched her go. Then he looked at me with the expression that meant he was deciding whether to say something.

He didn't say anything.

We moved toward the checkout.

We passed the candy aisle on the way to the checkout.

I stopped, took a Hershey bar from the rack and put it in the cart.

Paul looked at it, then he looked at me. I looked back at him. I could feel anger radiating from my eyes.

He didn't say anything.

Outside, the heat had thickened since we'd come in. Paul loaded the bags into the trunk. He came around to my side and opened the door. I got in.

He got in and started the engine.

"You could have said something," I said. "To Carol. You could have turned the conversation."

He was looking at the backup camera.

"You didn't."

"No," he eased out of the space. "I didn't."

I looked out the window.

"She was your friend," he said. "Not mine. I wasn't sure what to say."

CHAPTER 43
Wednesday, July 22

Paul still didn't go to work. I woke to find him sitting on the edge of the bed, fully dressed but motionless. Seven-thirty. He should have left an hour ago.

"You called in sick?" I pushed myself up. Paul never called in. Not for colds, not for migraines, not when his father died.

"Personal matter." His voice was flat.

He turned to look at me, and I saw that expression from when he'd almost told me something and stopped and put it off until "tomorrow."

Tomorrow is now.

"Paul, what's wrong?"

He stood, paced to the window, and came back. His right hand went into his pocket. Stayed there.

"I saw a doctor on Monday," he said. "In Little Rock."

I was confused. He'd been here with me on Monday. Then I understood. I asked, "What kind of doctor?"

"Neurologist."

My mind was whirling. *Had he spoken to a doctor about me? Why?*

I said, "The day you left for work early. —Why would you see a neurologist?"

He said, "A movement disorder specialist."

Paul pulled his right hand out of his pocket. Held it out. It trembled.

Not much. Barely visible. The stress tremor I'd been seeing for months.

"I've been having symptoms," he said quietly.

"More than the tremor?"

"Stiffness in my shoulder. My handwriting gets smaller—I noticed at work." He stared at his hand. "I thought it was stress. Watching you deal with this, worrying about you. I thought maybe I was just copying your symptoms somehow. Psychosomatic."

"You've had symptoms and didn't tell me?"

"Didn't want to worry you. You know. Dr. Patel said stress can make Parkinson's worse...I made an appointment three months ago. You know how long the wait is for neurology."

I did know. I waited six months to get into my first appointment with Dr. Patel.

"But you didn't tell me you made the appointment."

He sat down beside me. "What was I supposed to say? 'Hey, I think I might have Parkinson's too, but I won't know for three months.'? You're already dealing with so much. The medication's side effects. Your tremor is getting worse. That fall." His voice cracked. "I didn't want to add, 'Maybe I'm sick too,' on top of everything else. Not until I knew for sure."

How had I not seen it before? How had I missed this?

I thought of all the jars he'd opened for me and the way he would reach for my arm when I went down a flight of stairs.

He said, "That's why I left for the Finch project early."

I asked even though I already knew the answer. "What did the doctor say?"

He reached into his jacket and pulled out a folded piece of paper. He set it on the bed between us.

Neither of us touched it.

I stared at the paper.

Finally, I picked it up and unfolded it.

Carbidopa-Levodopa. 25-100. Half a pill daily for one week. Then half a pill three times a day for a week.

I didn't need to read the rest. I knew the routine, the gradual increase of levodopa until reaching one pill three times a day. Then check in with the doctor, to see if the dose is right or if an overnight pill needed to be added.

The paper fell from my hands.

"I have Parkinson's disease." He said it fast, like ripping off a bandage. "Late-onset. Both of us have it now."

The tears came before I could stop them. Paul pulled me against him, and we held each other.

"I'm sorry," he whispered into my hair. "I'm sorry I didn't tell you about the appointment. I kept hoping I was wrong."

I pulled back to look at him. His face was wet.

"I'm so sorry, Paul. I know the symptoms and didn't recognize it. Or maybe I did and didn't want to."

He said, "Who's going to take care of us?"

Paul had spent four years gradually increasing his caregiving, what I had begun to think of as management. Of course, that is what he would be worried about.

"We'll take care of each other."

We sat there on the bed, both of us trying not to fall apart completely.

"Did he tell you anything about what to expect? I know early onset is different from late, but I'm not sure how."

The doctor said that there's a chance I'll progress faster, but everyone is different. He also said that the risk of cognitive involvement is higher. He wants me to take B12 and consider getting B12 injections."

"Did he say anything about why?" I asked. "I mean, did you tell him I had it too? Two people in the same house?"

"He said it's unusual. Parkinson's isn't contagious. It could be genetic or environmental. He said, most of the time, no cause can be found."

CHAPTER 44

Wednesday, July 22

Paul moved heavily...the way he'd been moving all day, as if he were monitoring himself from a distance. Oil in the pan. Chicken from the package. He'd already wiped the counter twice without reason.

He said, "It suddenly feels real, now that I've told you."

The chicken began to sizzle. Paul stood over it, spatula in hand, not moving.

"You don't have to cook whenever you're home. I can cook for us."

He said, "I want to."

I thought I understood what he was feeling. He wanted to be the person he thought he was. There was a difference between wanting to cook and the feeling of being needed.

Is he performing capability, performing appetite?

I said, “On Saturday, something happened to me. I discovered that I’ve been reducing myself. I left behind parts of my life before Parkinson’s could steal more from me.”

He flipped the chicken. His hand shook, and he gripped the spatula harder, and it stilled again.

He has been dealing with this alone for months.

I didn't know whether to be furious, wrecked or simply sad for him.

We ate at the table because Paul had set it. It almost made me cry — Paul’s habit of infusing order in the middle of everything he was dealing with.

I broke the silence and said, “I think everyone responds to a diagnosis differently. Some people go into denial. Someone else might pretend that everything is normal. Some get angry. Some leave themselves behind before Parkinson’s has the power to take it from them. That’s sort of what I did. I think you’ll go through a process too. And you might not even know you went through an acceptance period until months or years later...I mean, I’m four years in and just coming to terms with it...I think.”

Paul didn’t respond for quite a while. Neither of us ate much. I pushed my food around my plate. Picked at the chicken.

“I had a whole spreadsheet,” Paul said. “For retirement. Which parks in what order? Acadia first, then down through the South, then west. I had the campgrounds picked out.”

I knew about the spreadsheet. I had teased him about it. “Only you,” I'd said, “would put a spreadsheet between you and a sunset.”

Today, that spreadsheet represented more than taking trips. It spoke of a lost future.

We can still travel," I said, and heard how hollow my words were even before he looked at me.

He said, "When you were diagnosed, I knew that the retirement plan would never happen. Because I had to take care of you…and you…you wouldn't be hiking trails or bungee jumping."

"Bungee jumping? Really? I never thought of you doing that. But I can travel. Having Parkinson's doesn't stop me from traveling. It doesn't need to stop you."

He set down his fork. "I'm supposed to be at the finish line of everything I've built. The career. The plans. Finally getting to use what we saved." He looked at his hands on the table. "We were supposed to have good years ahead. That was the whole idea."

"I know."

"That's gone now." He said it quietly. Not angry. "Whatever I thought was coming — that's gone."

I've spent years grieving my future alone, not wanting to make Paul carry it too. He's been doing the same thing. We've been grieving separately, in the same house, in the same bed, grieving alone to protect each other.

Eventually, we left our plates on the table and moved to the living room. Paul sat on the couch. I sat beside him.

"The doctor asked if I'd had thoughts of not being here," Paul said.

"What did you tell him?"

"I said no." He paused. "That wasn't entirely true."

I waited.

"Not seriously," he said. "Nothing like a plan. Just the thought that it might be easier. To not have to watch myself become someone who can't function."

"I know that thought," I said.

He looked at me.

"It comes at night sometimes. One morning I had the thought before my first pill. I wondered, what if I just didn't take the pill? What if I just stopped living?" I kept my voice even. "It doesn't stay. But it comes."

"Yeah."

"Does it scare you?"

He thought about it. "It scares me that it doesn't scare me more."

I understood that exactly. *The thought arrives flat, almost practical, when I'm exhausted or before I am awake enough to feel its weight. It doesn't feel like a crisis, just calculation. Not caring either way, about living or not, is an aspect of Parkinson's no one told me about.*

I moved closer to him on the couch.

"I talked to someone," I said. "When it got bad last spring. A therapist who works with chronic illness patients."

"Did it help?"

I thought about how to answer honestly. "It made the feeling smaller. Less like a fact." I looked at him.

He nodded slowly. Not a commitment. Just receiving it.

My phone buzzed on the cushion beside me. Rebecca. She wrote, 'Missed seeing you yesterday. Hope everything is alright."

I looked at the message for a long moment.

Three months ago, I would have ignored the message. I knew that version of myself intimately — the one who kept contracting, who made her circle smaller, who called retreat self-care and called disappearing rest.

I was still that person, but I could feel the person I was before I was diagnosed with Parkinson's. I wanted to be her again.

I typed back, "I'll be there."

I sent it before I could think too much.

Paul was watching me.

"Support group," I said.

He nodded. Something moved across his face — not quite relief, not quite hope. Recognition, maybe. His wife, still here. Still choosing.

I said, "You should come too."

"Maybe."

"Paul," I said it gently. "You can't engineer your way out of this one."

He laughed — short, surprised, real. The first real laugh of the day. It changed his whole face.

"No," he said. "I really can't."

CHAPTER 45

Sunday, July 26

We had been careful with each other for days. Not cold. Not distant. The carefulness of people navigating something fragile — moving past each other in the kitchen with extra space, asking before touching, making the small adjustments that accumulate when both people in a room are afraid of being the one who breaks something.

Sunday evening, Paul came to bed before ten. This was unusual. Paul's version of early was eleven, unless he fell asleep on the couch. He stood in the doorway in his undershirt and looked at the bed, and then at me, and then at the book I wasn't reading.

I looked back at him over it. "What?"

"Nothing." He came in and sat on his side and took his watch off and set it on the nightstand the way he always did.

I put the book down.

Sex had become infrequent over the last two years.

I reasoned with myself that some of the loss of interest was from aging. I knew that some of it was from Parkinson's apathy and fatigue. Mostly, I no longer trusted that my body wouldn't embarrass me.

Paul had learned not to start because I often refused. He had adjusted to my leaving this part of our marriage.

He turned off the lamp and lay down facing me in the dark. His hand found my arm and stayed there, just present, not asking anything. I could feel the slight tremor in his fingers. I had felt it for months without letting myself feel it, and now I felt it.

I moved closer.

What followed was not graceful. It had not been graceful for some time. But this was more awkward than usual, complicated by the weight of knowing Paul's diagnosis.

There was a moment when we had to stop and reorient, which neither of us commented on, a practice we had become accustomed to. His body and my body, both imperfect, both present.

Midway through, my leg cramped. Not a subtle cramp. The kind that required stopping entirely while I sat up and pressed my heel down against the mattress and breathed through it with my jaw set. He sat up beside me and waited. The cramp moved through and released. I sat there for a moment in the dark.

I said, "I'm sorry."

He was quiet for a moment. He shifted back toward me. Not with urgency — just returning to where we had been, which felt like its own kind of decision. We found our way back, slower, differently than we had started, neither performing anything for the other.

It was not what it used to be. It was also not what it had been for the last two years — the carefully managed movement that might culminate in reward. This was something else. Bodies that were telling the truth about themselves. Two people in the same dark, inside the same life, both knowing what the other knew. It was better than we'd known in years.

Afterwards, we lay still for a while.

The window was open. The neighborhood was doing what it did at this hour.

"I keep thinking about the spreadsheet," Paul said to the ceiling.

"Which one?"

"The one from before. The parks. Acadia. The whole itinerary." He was quiet for a moment. "I had us visit twenty-two national parks in four years."

I looked at the ceiling with him.

"We could still go," I said.

He didn't answer.

I said, "It doesn't need to be all twenty-two."

We just lay there, holding each other as the ceiling fan turned.

I said, “We could go to Acadia. One Park. A hotel. We could watch the sunrise from the top of a mountain. You would tell me the geological history of the formation, and I would pretend to listen.”

He made a sound. Not quite a laugh. Something adjacent.

“You'd be asleep before sunrise,” he said.

“I'd make the effort.”

He said, “You'd fall asleep in the car on the way up.”

“And you'd wake me up anyway because you would need someone to talk to about the sunrise.”

“Okay,” he said. “Acadia.”

His hand found mine between us in the dark. Not the checking hold — not him steadying me. Just two hands...two warm hands...understanding each other in a way we hadn’t before.

CHAPTER 46

Tuesday, July 28

By Tuesday morning, I was grieving something I couldn't name. Not his diagnosis — that grief was clear and had an address. This was something else...something that had arrived quietly in the days since Paul told me. His diagnosis had settled into the house.

I watched Paul iron his shirt.

The diagnosis was still new enough to have the quality of a wound. His boss had said, "Take whatever time you need." His sister had called twice. There was a casserole in our refrigerator from a neighbor who didn't know him well enough to know he didn't eat casserole.

A whole apparatus of concern had assembled itself around him.

My diagnosis was four years old. I knew what that meant. My diagnosis was now invisible, absorbed, replaced by the normalcy of living. It meant that the crisis had passed — not because things were better. I had never returned to *fine,* despite years of saying, "I'm fine." I had learned to manage the absence of *getting better* so efficiently that when symptoms got worse, they didn't read as an emergency from the outside.

Paul had built accommodation into our life so well that most days neither of us had to look directly at what we were accommodating. The coffee table was against the wall. The rug was gone. There was a night light in the hall. And most recently, Paul *improved* the bathroom and kitchen. He even added a ramp leading to our front door. The whole invisible architecture of life had been reorganized around what I could no longer do or what might happen in the future.

And now he had Parkinson's too.

I had spent years being a patient. I was the one that the house was organized around. I was the one Paul watched from doorways with careful, unannounced attention.

That role cost me. I was only now understanding this, only now that it was shifting. But it had been the structure I lived in for years. I was the sick one. Take that away and I didn't yet know what was left, who I was in our marriage—now that we were both patients and I was rebelling against being managed. *Am I to be Paul's caregiver?*

This morning, I wasn't grieving his diagnosis. I was grieving the role I'd never chosen and had somehow come to need. I was grieving the invisibility of having done Parkinson's longer.

The thing I couldn't look at directly, what I kept approaching and turning away from — was fear. Not of his Parkinson's disease...of what I already knew, and he didn't yet...the road that lay ahead of him, which I had already walked further down, and which I knew did not get easier in the ways he would want it to.

Paul put his shirt on and started buttoning it from the bottom.

He used to start from the top.

He didn't notice until the fourth button. Then he stopped. He looked down at his own chest with an expression I hadn't seen before — not frustration, something quieter, a man taking inventory of a system that had changed its operating behavior — and unbuttoned the shirt and started again from the top, without comment.

I watched this from the doorway.

"You've said it twice since breakfast," he said without looking up.

"I haven't said anything."

"You said, 'The discussion there is raw. Are you sure you want to come?' and just now with your face." He examined the shirt collar. "I'm aware of what a support group involves. I have Parkinson's. The venue is correct."

I crossed the room and stood behind him and put my hands on his shoulders and looked at both of us in the mirror. He looked up and met my eyes in the glass. Neither of us said anything. I watched him finish his last button, his hands steadier now, thanks to levodopa, or maybe I was just imagining the difference.

I said, “Good. I’m proud of you. Ready?”

He nodded. Put his hand over mine. Suddenly, I wished we were staying home...reliving our time together last night and the night before.

CHAPTER 47

Tuesday, July 28

The drive took eleven minutes. I know because Paul counted. He'd started timing things—durations, distances, and how long it took for his medication to kick-in. I used to do that too. I believed that "being on" would eventually become predictable. It had for a short time and then it totally changed. I hadn't told him yet because he was still new to Parkinson's and some things you had to arrive at yourself.

The center's parking lot was half-full. I got out before he came around to my side. Paul took my elbow. A week ago, he would have taken my hand.

He's already adjusting himself, even before his symptoms demand change. He's doing what I did.

I didn't know yet whether the change in how he conducted himself was devastating or was simply practical. *Perhaps it's what sometimes happens when the diagnosis lands and has not yet been fully understood, integrated, or accepted.*

CHAPTER 48

Tuesday, July 28

Room 107. The burned-coffee smell hit before the door fully opened—that scorched note that had become, somehow, a smell associated with being understood. The sign still had the smudge across its exclamation point.

Gerald was already there. His phone was out. Gerald squinted at it.

Diane sat beside him, with her needles going. This week's project appeared to be a gray mystery that was already showing dropped stitches near the bottom right corner.

Martin sat with his legs extended. He was speaking with Elizabeth, who sat beside David at their habitual angle. Her shoulder almost touched David's.

Robert kept his cane across his knees. He was sitting beside Linda.

Tom's wheelchair was near the window. Sarah was close but not touching, her shoulder nearly at his ear. When she looked up and saw Paul, her eyes moved over him the way you assess a room for exits—not unkindly, functionally. The assessment of someone who has learned to read new arrivals for their distance from the shore.

Rebecca gave me a small nod and smile that said, you came back. She looked at Paul and tilted her head. I hadn't yet told her about Paul's diagnosis.

Michelle sat with the soles of her running shoes pressed to the floor, like she needed to feel the contact. I wondered, *is she creating a new version of herself…one where she leaves her old life or embracing a new way of living it?*

We took two chairs near Rebecca. Paul sat beside me and folded his hands. I knew what he was going through, sitting here for the first time.

Linda moved to the center of the circle. She had the competence of someone who had learned to hold a room without controlling it.

"Good morning." She paused briefly, glancing at Paul. "I hope everyone has had a good week. Let's get started. Jump in when you're ready. Who wants to start?"

"I will. I think a lot of my life is performed. Even parts that have nothing to do with Parkinson's," Gerald said, not looking up from his phone. "Half of us spent the drive here performing. I performed confidence at a traffic light and pulled something in my shoulder."

Two people laughed. Diane's needles kept clicking.

"Who are you now?" Linda said. She sat down.

The room was quiet.

"Smaller," Diane said, without looking up from the gray thing in her lap.

Nobody laughed.

"I was a runner," Michelle said. "Five mornings a week. Before coffee, before my kids were up. Running was mine. The one thing nobody could ask me to share." She looked at her shoes. "I can't run like I used to. My gaits off. And I know it sounds small—my husband says it's small. 'Just walk,' he says. But it wasn't running. It was who I was while I ran. That version of me...is it disappearing? I don't know what's there instead. So, I've been sleeping until seven and telling myself that running is a choice."

The room received this without comment.

"I was a contractor," Gerald said. Not to Michelle—just in parallel, the way Gerald answered questions on his own track. "Thirty-one years. Built houses. My hands—" he looked at them, "—I could feel a quarter-inch variance. Tell by touch whether a joint was true." He turned his phone face-down on his knee. "My son runs the business now. He calls to ask my opinion. He doesn't need my opinion. He's better than I was at thirty-nine. But he calls."

There was something about Gerald's sentences. They always ended up somewhere quieter than where they started. You'd brace for the blunt thing, and the blunt thing would turn out to have a different inside.

"I'm still a pharmacist," Rebecca said. "I still go to work. But I check my hands before work every day and wonder."

“What happens if the tremor gets worse or stays?” Linda asked.

Rebecca was quiet for a moment. “I don't know,” she said. “I'm hoping I never find out.”

“My new now is my face.” We waited for Elizabeth to take a breath. “I practice...facial expressions,” Elizabeth said. She rarely spoke. When she did, people listened not from courtesy but because of the quality of what she had to say. She waited until the right moment to speak, with the patience of someone who had learned that waiting was itself a skill.

“The mask,” she said. Her voice was barely above a whisper. “It takes the face. Not all at once. Bit by bit. The muscles—” she stopped. Started again. “You stop looking the way you feel...People think you're angry...Or far away. They stop—including you.”

Her son David said, “I didn't know that.”

Elizabeth looked at him. “I know you didn't.” One breath. “That was the point.”

Something passed between them that the room didn't examine.

I thought about my own morning diagnostic: check the tremor, see if I had started developing the mask, assess which tells I could hide and which I'd have to carry openly today. I'd been calling it “getting dressed.”

I was surprised when I heard Paul speaking.

“I can't tell anymore,” he said. “When am I performing? I can't find the seam.” He looked up slowly. “I recently found out I have Parkinson's. I told my wife about a week later. Before that, I spent six months explaining things away. I knew exactly how to do—distraction, anything to avoid worrying Joy.” He paused. “I guess I have a sophisticated and long-practiced talent for lying to myself about things I don't want to be true.”

“That's not unusual here,” Rebecca said. She glanced over at me.

“It’s easier to blame other things. Because Parkinson’s is too expensive,” Diane said. Her needles paused, just for a moment. “Not financially. Just—everything it would cost you to let it be true.”

Paul nodded slowly.

I watched him and felt the thing I'd been circling all morning resolve into words. He had spent months on the outside of this disease—managing me, watching for signs of his own, thinking about the infrastructure of our adjusted life. And now he was inside Parkinson’s, hearing and finally understanding things I had tried to tell him but could only reach you by living inside Parkinson’s.

“What did you think it was?” Robert asked Paul.

“Fear,” Paul said. “I thought I was scared about Joy. About work. I thought the tremor was my body expressing what I couldn't say.” He glanced at me. “I wondered if I was unconsciously copying Joy. And it was like, sometimes, all I could see of Joy was her disease. I love her but the idea of being her caregiver. Sometimes it was too much.”

Diane said, “Like the disease and the person aren't separate things. You’re not just Parkinson's. You're Paul, who also has Parkinson's.”

CHAPTER 49

Tuesday, July 28

Sarah broke during the break. Not dramatically—it was too small and too practiced for drama. She'd gone to refill Tom's water, and she stood at the table with her back to the room. I watched her press the heel of her hand against her sternum. One breath. Two. She picked up the cup, turned around, and her face was arranged.

Nobody else saw. Or nobody said anything.

That is what eight years looks like from inside Parkinson's. Not Tom in the wheelchair, the ramp, or the schedule organized around medication windows. Sarah at the water table, holding herself together with one hand pressed to her chest, and then returning.

I have been doing that too. Not as long. Not as well. But I have been doing that.

I hadn't told Paul that I was angry. Not for anything he'd done, for the fact that he got to walk into this disease fresh. My grief had edges worn down, smoothed by time. His experience still had sharp corners on it. That wasn't his fault. It was wrong to be angry about it. But it was true.

I wouldn't say it today. But I was going to have to tell Paul eventually, because years of not saying true things had built up pressure.

Paul had gotten coffee. He came back with two cups, handed me one, tasted his own. He said, "You weren't exaggerating."

"I never exaggerate about coffee."

He drank it anyway. That was Paul: identify the problem precisely, register the objection formally, adapt without fuss. I was starting to understand that this might become his relationship with Parkinson's too. I couldn't decide yet whether that would save us both or make me want to put something through a wall.

Michelle had brought cookies. Homemade chocolate chip, dark at the edges. Gerald had eaten three before anyone else finished their first. Diane glared at him. Gerald glared back.

"I have Parkinson's," Gerald said. "I'm seizing the moment."

"That expression refers to opportunities," Diane said. "Not baked goods."

"I've redefined it. For personal use." He took a fourth cookie and set it on his knee with the precision of a man making a formal claim.

Diane's needles kept going. The gray thing was developing a noticeable lean toward its left side. She appeared not to notice, or to mind.

The cookie was excellent. Michelle looked surprised and grateful when I said so. She baked them, she told me, when she couldn't sleep.

Linda settled back in her chair, and the room settled with her. She had a quality I'd noticed from the beginning. She could redirect a room without announcing the turn. You were always somewhere new before you noticed you were moving.

"The small losses," she said. "Not the diagnosis. Not the ones that make the formal list of symptoms. The ones that happen in the ordinary minutes of a day and don't warrant a doctor's appointment. They don't fit into what people mean when they ask how you're doing." She looked around the circle. "What are you losing that nobody asks about?"

"Spontaneity," Michelle said. "I can't do anything on impulse anymore. Everything runs through the same calculation: when did I take my last dose, what's the terrain like, how far is the parking, where's the bathroom. My husband wants to stop somewhere on the way home, and I must stop and compute. He thinks I don't want to go. I want to go. I just need the timing to be right, and he can't see that those are different things."

"The planning is exhausting," Jennifer said. "It's not the going. It's the before-the-going and the collapse afterwards. By the time I've decided to go somewhere, I've already spent what going there would have cost."

Rebecca said. "Someone asked me a small scheduling question. I stood there for a good minute unable to begin an answer. They thought I was distracted. I was depleted. That's a different thing entirely."

"Sixteen years of fatigue," Diane confirmed.

Paul made a small sound. He didn't know yet what it cost to negotiate with the disease. The loneliness of being the first to see the difference and having nowhere to put the seeing. *I'm glad he is here.*

Gerald said, "When I stop being angry at accommodation and start only being grateful, I think that's when I'll call it quits. But I have a shower chair now. I named him."

"What's its name?" Michelle asked.

"Gerald Junior," he said.

The room laughed—the real kind, that surfaces from somewhere genuine rather than being produced for the occasion.

"We moved the coffee table," I said.

Everyone looked at me.

I said, "It's for traffic flow." I paused. "Our good dishes are on a lower shelf, so I don't have to reach." I looked at the floor. "The house is reorganizing itself around Parkinson's. And I understand it. I appreciate it. But sometimes I walk through the living room and miss how the house used to feel."

Paul was listening. He nodded.

"We have a ramp," Sarah had been quiet since the break. She was looking at Tom—not at us—with an expression that was completely composed.

"Over the front steps." Sarah added, "The ramp means Tom can get outside without it being an operation. Last week, he sat outside by himself for two hours."

She was still looking at Tom. "I sat inside by myself. It was nice."

Tom said something I couldn't understand. She didn't look at him.

"Can I say something?" Paul asked.

"Of course," Linda said.

"I built all of it," he said. "The accommodations. I tied Joy's shoes." He smiled at me. "I thought that was what love looked like. Making the adaptation invisible so she didn't have to acknowledge what life was changing. Taking some of the weight so she didn't have to carry it."

He squeezed my hand and said, "Now I understand that I was solving problems before there was a problem. I didn't let her ask for help. I thought I was protecting her. I think I was also protecting myself."

"That's how it goes," Sarah said.

"My wife carries my toolbox," Gerald said to Paul. "Every time I want to take my tools somewhere, she carries them. I never asked her to. I don't want her to."

Gerald looked at Paul steadily. "First time she did it, I wanted to take it back. Now I'll hold the door while she carries it. It's not what I'd have chosen. But holding the door is not nothing. It's what I've got, so I made it something."

Paul said, "I've been the one who carried the toolbox." He didn't look at me. "I'm going to have to let Joy carry mine."

"You're going to hate it," Gerald said.

CHAPTER 50

Tuesday, July 28

"There are days," Linda said, "when you look at the life you're managing, and you ask whether it's worth managing. Not a crisis. Not the edge. The days when the weight of it is simply visible and you try to make the arithmetic work. Maybe it doesn't." She looked around the circle. "I'm not asking who's in danger. I'm asking who recognizes what I'm describing."

Robert's hand went up. Jennifer's. Martin's. Diane's, her needles going still for a breath before resuming. Michelle's—hesitant, then certain. The woman on four medications, looking at the carpet. Sarah's raised hand arrived differently than the others. She had organized everything around Tom's life continuing.

Paul and I looked at each other and raised our hands.

"Those days are real," Linda said. "They're the days when the weight is visible. But a day when the weight is visible is not the same as a day when you've stopped believing you can carry it. One is part of living with this. The other is more than this room." She paused. "What gets people through the first kind?"

"Spite," Gerald said.

Everyone looked at him and erupted in laughter.

"I mean it. A doctor described my future to me and I decided then. Hell no." Gerald paused. "My brother-in-law asked if I'd considered assisted living. I was standing in his kitchen, holding a beer. Without assistance." He crossed his arms. "I get out of bed some mornings because I intend to outlast what those people think."

Linda said, "This disease wants people to put their lives on hold."

Paul let go of my hand to rub the back of his neck.

Nobody said anything.

"How do you not hate the life you got instead of the one you planned?" Paul asked.

"Some days I do hate it," Diane said. "There's no moral requirement to make your peace with this. The hate is real, and it's allowed. I hate Parkinson's."

Gerald said, very quietly for Gerald: "Same."

Rebecca nodded.

I looked at Paul beside me. He couldn't save me from this disease. I couldn't save him. But we could stay. We could be in the same room with it, without managing each other's share of hating it. That was different from saving.

When Linda closed the meeting, Sarah stopped in front of Paul. She said, "You're allowed to be exactly where you are."

I watched her take the wheelchair handles and move Tom toward the door.

Rebecca sat beside me while the room emptied. "Same time next week?"

I looked at Paul. He was watching Sarah navigate the door.

"Yes," he said, still watching Sarah. "Same time."

The parking lot was hot.

"I kept thinking I needed to understand why," Paul said. "Why both of us? Why now? I kept thinking if I could locate the cause I could—" He stopped. "Do something with it. File it somewhere. Make it make sense."

"I know."

"But sitting in that room." He was quiet for a moment. "Nobody in that room was asking why anymore. They were just living in the question of how. How to carry it. How to stay."

"That's the only question, isn't it?"

Paul opened my door.

"We take turns carrying it," I said as I got in. "When you can't, I carry more. When I can't, you do. We can stop deciding what the other one can handle."

Paul got in and said, "Maybe we'll go see all twenty-two national parks, after all."

CHAPTER 51

Wednesday, August 5

The cathedral in my dream had no builder. I understood this, as though the fact was woven through the dream. The walls rose on both sides, stone. It carried centuries of weather and candlelight and the breath of people praying. The walls rose and rose and at some point, simply stopped being walls and became sky. The transition was so gradual it was impossible to locate.

The floor was water. Not flooded — the water was the floor, perfectly level, perfectly still, clear down to the stone beneath it. I looked down through the water at my feet. I was standing on the water, not in the water. I understood that I needed to see what was under the water. I bent down.

The water came up my wrists. It had no temperature. I put my palms on the stone floor beneath me and felt the texture of what was there.

The stone reminded me of braille, each bump and curve seemed purposeful. I knew the stone texture carried meaning.

I looked closer.

The floor was covered in letters that were present in the stone, the way grain was present in wood. It was as though the stone had always contained letters, and the water had simply made them visible.

I tried to read them.

They were in no alphabet I recognized. The letters appeared to be something that existed before language organized itself into the forms I knew.

My right hand moved. I watched it the way I sometimes watched my hand during waking hours — with the attention of a person observing something that belonged to her and operated independently.

My fingers traced the letters I couldn't read. When I traced, the letters became briefly luminous — not bright, the luminosity of things seen at the edge of vision, present when you didn't look directly, gone when you did. I understood, without being able to say how I understood, that this was not a message. The letters were not trying to tell me something I didn't know.

They were simply showing me what had always been there. Underneath everything. Prior to everything. They were waiting, with patience.

CHAPTER 52

Wednesday, August 5

Paul's voice came through the dream like a hand reaching into water, touching mine. "Joy. Joy."

I was still tracing. My right hand moved across the stone floor of the cathedral, the letters lighting and going dark. The water was around our hands. Paul's voice echoed in the cathedral. The cathedral was shaking, as some outside force was rending the water from the floor, wall from ceiling. I looked at a wall, our bedroom arriving in pieces, the familiar dark rectangle of it, the curtains, the pale shape of the window.

I was lying on my side facing away from Paul and my right arm was extended fully in front of me, reaching, my hand open. I had been moving it — I could feel the motion still in my arm, the ghost of the gesture, the memory of reaching for something across a floor that wasn't there.

Paul's hand was on my shoulder. "Hey," he said. "Hey. Come back."

I pulled my arm in and assembled the room around me. “How long,” I said.

“Few minutes.” He paused. “You were reaching for something.”

“I remember.”

“Did you get it?”

“I don't know,” I said. “Sorry, I woke you.”

Paul moved closer. “Was it the bad kind?” Paul asked.

“No.”

He was quiet. His hand was still moving, slow, against my back.

“I was somewhere,” I said. “I was reading something. With my hand.” I paused. “I couldn't understand it. But I understood it was there.”

The current from the dream was still moving through my chest — not a thought about it, not a memory of it, the thing itself, steady and unhurried, passing through the way light passed through the open top of the cathedral, without needing to arrive anywhere, without needing to be named.

Paul's breathing deepened. His hand stilled on my back, heavy now with sleep.

CHAPTER 53

Thursday, August 20

Paul had been in his office since seven. He wasn't working — I could tell by the silence. When Paul worked, the house had a sound: the low tap of keys, the periodic roll of his chair, the sound of him getting up to look at something on the wall and sitting back down.

I drank my coffee at the kitchen table. I had gotten better at not going to check on him, which was itself a form of progress that no one would ever congratulate me for.

A couple hours later, he came out.

He was dressed and looked like he was going somewhere.

"I need to tell you something," he said.

"Okay."

He came to the table and sat down across from me. He looked at the table for a moment, then at his hands, then at me. The gesture seemed like a sequence of a man trying to locate a thing that isn't where he usually keeps things.

“I've been talking to Richards,” he said.

I waited.

“About the Finch project. About — my capacity. Going forward.”

I nodded.

“He's been patient. He's kept the position open. But he thinks I should take more time. I think he means permanently.”

“What do you think?”

He said, “I've been compensating. For — a while.” He said it flat.

“I can't do the work. Not the way it needs to be done.” He paused. “I can't do what needs done anymore. I can see part of it. Pieces. But the whole — I lose it. I'll be in the middle of a calculation, and the thread goes.”

“Paul,” I said. “What do you want to do?”

“I want to stop,” he said. “I want to stop before—” He stopped. Pressed his lips together. Started again. “I want to leave while it is still my choice.”

“Then stop. Call Richards today. Tell him you're not coming back.” I kept my voice steady. Not because it was easy. Because he needed steady right now. “You decided. That's done.”

“There are things to figure out,” he said. “Practical things.”

“We'll figure them out.”

"I had plans for this period. Finch would have been the last major project before I scaled back. I had...I had a whole sequence mapped. It doesn't look like my plan is going to work."

"No."

He said, "I thought I'd have more time."

I didn't say anything. There was nothing to say about it. I had thought that too, in a different context, four years ago, and the thought had not changed what was true.

He was quiet for a moment. "I'll call Richards this morning."

"Okay."

"I'll need some time. Alone. Would you mind?"

"I'll go out," I said. "I need to pick up a few things. I'll be back by lunch."

He nodded.

At the door I stopped.

"Paul."

He looked up.

"You're more than an engineer."

He smiled.

CHAPTER 54

Thursday, August 20

Paul was at the kitchen table when I came in.

"Done?"

He said, "I'm officially retired."

I put the grocery bags on the counter. He didn't move to help, which I registered and did not remark on.

"How did it go?"

"Fine. He was decent about it. He offered severance above what he had to." Paul looked at his blue cup. "He said it had been a privilege to work with me."

Something moved in his face when he said that. The word *privilege* landed. I watched it move through him and settle.

"It was," I said. "A privilege."

He looked at me.

"For them," I said. "You were very good at it."

His jaw shifted. The slight compression of a man who will not cry in his own kitchen on a Thursday morning, who has given himself exactly this much room and will not take more.

"Yes," he said. "I was."

I put the kettle on and hand-washed a new cup. The cup was stoneware, a muted slate blue — not the bright flag blue of his maple leaf mug, but something quieter, like water under cloud cover. It was wide at the base, slightly narrower at the rim. Heavy enough that you knew it was there when you picked it up. The cup was uneven in the way of handmade things, darker in the grooves, lighter where the clay rose. It didn't have a handle. You could wrap both hands around it.

He sat at the kitchen table, and I stood at the counter making tea we didn't need.

The kettle boiled. I poured two cups and set one in front of him. He noticed. Not immediately. First, he just received it, the way you receive anything set in front of you when you're somewhere else in your mind. His hands went around it automatically.

He turned the cup slightly with both hands and felt the unevenness under his thumbs. It took a moment, and then he understood the new cup's purpose.

"This is a good cup." He drank his tea.

CHAPTER 55

Tuesday, August 25

The room smelled the same. Burned coffee, the scorch of a pot that had been sitting too long. I said, "It always smells like burned coffee here."

Paul said, "I don't smell anything."

We had usual chairs now. That had happened without discussion. Last week, Gerald had said, "It's simple. You sit somewhere twice and then it's yours."

Gerald was already there. He looked up when we came in, nodded at Paul with the nod of men who have sat in the same circle long enough to have developed a shorthand.

Diane had turned-in her yarn and replaced it with a sketching pad and pencils. Her current project was a deep charcoal gray. I caught a glimpse of her drawing. It appeared to be a highly detailed flower.

Rebecca came in behind us. She caught my eye and held it for a moment. We had gone out for lunch many times, including several returns to the Corner Café.

Martin came in quietly and took his usual chair, touching his head briefly as he sat — the DBS scar, the gesture so habitual he probably didn't know he still made it.

Sarah and Tom always sat near the window. She looked up when we entered. Her eyes moved to Paul. She smiled. She admitted to me once that she felt Paul could understand something of her life the rest of us couldn't.

Linda came in, set her things down, looked around the circle silently taking attendance not by name but by faces.

"We have someone joining us today," she said. "First time. But I expect she won't be here until we've started. I think we will—"

The door opened.

I recognized her before she had fully entered. The posture first, then her face. It was Dr. Patel. Her white coat had been replaced with jeans and a pretty short-sleeved shirt. Her hair was down. She found an empty chair.

Linda said, "And our new person is here. Why don't you introduce yourself. Then we'll get started."

"I'm Tara," she said. "I was diagnosed in February."

"Hi, Tara," Gerald said. "Welcome to the Coffee Club."

Several of us laughed. Linda said, "We probably should get a good coffee maker and maybe a name. I'll ensure better coffee next week. Gerald, maybe you could think of a good name?"

Gerald smiled.

Linda looked around the circle. “Last week we discussed some clinical trials and current treatment options. I hope everyone enjoyed our guest speaker. Today’s question is, what have you stopped admitting you want?”

“Not what you've accepted,” Linda said. “Not what you've made peace with. What do you want but you to stopped letting yourself want?”

No one answered.

Linda said, “Whatever it is. What have you stopped admitting?”

“I want to drive,” Robert said. He said it quietly. We all knew Robert had given up driving a month ago. He had mentioned it once, sideways, in the context of something else. He had never said it directly until now.

“Not far. Not on a highway. I want to drive to the hardware store on Saturday morning. The way I drove to the hardware store for forty years.” He looked at his cane across his knees. “Without asking anyone for permission. I want to be the person who just goes.”

“I want my husband to look at me...the way...he looked at me...before,” Elizabeth said. Her voice was louder than it had been. It was still breathy, but it was easier to hear her.

Linda said, “Elizabeth, you sound good. We can hear you without trying.”

“Thank you. I’ve been doing Speak Out.”

“I want to stop waiting to feel ready,” Rebecca said.

“I want to stop being afraid of what I know,” Paul said.

"That takes a while," Gerald said. "I'm still afraid. Linda, I think for a while I thought I wasn't allowed to want some things."

Linda said, "Like what?"

Gerald said, "I want to get on a plane and go visit my son. I know it won't happen. But I thought it was wrong to even want it. Now I know it's alright to want things like that."

"I want to know," Tara said, "whether I have been helping people or just medicating them."

Gerald laughed. "Are you a drug dealer?"

"I'm a doctor. I've delivered this diagnosis more times than I can count."

Rebecca said, "I'm a pharmacist and I use Levodopa. I know the side effects and benefits. You raise a good question, Tara."

Tara said, "When I was practicing, I often felt frustrated by the limits of what I could offer my patients. Now I'm more than frustrated. I'm angry."

CHAPTER 56

Tuesday, August 25

Linda's question about *wanting* had done its work. *Wanting* had moved through the circle and left me carrying something I hadn't quite named before.

Michelle said. "Tara. I hope it's alright if I ask you a question. Maybe I'm asking everyone. I know levodopa is the answer. I know that's what I'm supposed to take." She stopped. Started again. "What if I want to know who I am without the medication, just — you know, in my body, whether I'm still here? The before person. The one who's mine." She looked up. "Is that allowed?"

Rebecca said, "Levodopa doesn't slow Parkinson's. It can help with the tremor."

"The medication didn't make me disappear," Diane said. "I have more energy, I think."

Rebecca surprised me. She said, "It makes me sleepy sometimes. When I first started using it, I felt slightly high. Whenever my dose is increased, I have that mildly high feeling."

"Joy has been thinking about it too," Paul said.

The room turned toward us.

"She's been thinking about coming off the medication. We've talked about it. At home." He looked around the circle. "I don't think she should."

The room held this without taking sides.

"Paul," I said.

"I know." He looked at me. "I know this isn't the place. But it came up." He squeezed my hand. "I'm saying it because I'm afraid. I've watched you and I know what the medication gives you. I'm afraid of what happens if it's not there." Paul looked at my hands. "I know the levodopa has helped me. And you're further along than I am."

I said, "I've built the person I am now. Built myself around managing Parkinson's. I've gotten good at it. I've learned what the medication gives me and I've learned to work within the on times." I looked at Paul. "But I'm not sure I want to live this way, following the clock of on and off."

"What if being off levodopa is worse?" he said.

"Then I'll know. And knowing will be better than not knowing."

"That's not always true," Paul said.

Owen said, "Can I say something that might be uncomfortable?"

"That's generally what we do here," Gerald said.

"I came here because my neurologist referred me. I've been coming for two months, and it helps." He paused. "But I want to ask something honestly. Are we helping each other live better, or are we helping each other accept less life?"

Owen looked around the circle. "Because I hear a lot of talk in this room about acceptance and adaptation and making peace. I'm two months into this diagnosis. I'm not ready to make peace. I want to fight this. I want to try every experimental treatment. I want to be aggressive." He made a fist. "Sometimes I'm sitting here and feel like that is wrong somehow. Like I'm not doing Parkinson's right."

Gerald was looking at Owen steadily.

Owen said, "Levodopa is a way to fight."

"You're not wrong," Gerald said. "Two months in, you fight. That's correct. That's what two months in looks like." Gerald cleared his throat. "Seven years in, you still fight. Just differently. You learn what's worth the energy, and you put it there." He turned his coffee cup. "The acceptance isn't giving up. It's redirecting and choosing how to fight." He drank. Made a face. "I'm still mad about the coffee."

Two people laughed.

Rebecca leaned forward slightly. "The experimental treatments — some of them are real. Some are desperation dressed as hope. Learning to tell the difference isn't giving up. It's how you stay in the fight." She looked at Owen. "And you probably can't tell the difference alone. You need people who've been in this longer." She looked at Dr. Patel. "Knowledgeable doctors. Medical journals. And people who will support you in fighting it. That's what this room is for."

Dr. Tara Patel was holding herself stiffly in her chair. She caught me looking at her. She didn't look away. Neither did I.

CHAPTER 57

Wednesday, August 26

The coffee shop was Paul's idea, offered the way he offered things now — not with a plan already made, but with a question underneath the question: *Can we still do this?*

The place was narrow and deep, its furniture accumulated over years rather than chosen — mismatched chairs, a long wooden counter worn pale where elbows had rested. It smelled of espresso and cardamom, and the noise of the morning moved through it the way water moves through a stream. A woman in the corner typed without looking at her hands.

We found a table near the back. Paul pulled out my chair. He went to the counter, and I watched him take his place in line behind a young woman with long black hair. The young woman ordered without looking up. The server was already moving before she finished.

Paul reached the counter.

"What can I get you?"

Paul looked at the board. He had been drinking the same coffee since before we married: black, medium roast, heavy sugar. The server waited.

"Medium roast," he said. "Black." He paused one beat too long. His gaze drifted back to the board. "The tea. Chai."

He knew I drank chai. He had ordered it for me hundreds of times without consulting a menu.

He brought the cups to the table, set mine in front of me, and sat down. When he released his cup, his right hand trembled, and the ceramic made a small sound against the saucer.

I wrapped both hands around my cup.

"Busy," he said, looking at the room.

A bus went past the window, its shadow crossing the glass in one slow sweep.

"I've been thinking about Acadia," Paul said.

"We said in one year. September."

His eyes went to the middle distance — not to the window, not to me. His lips pressed together once. A breath in. The espresso machine behind the counter ran its cycle and finished. Paul was still somewhere inside whatever was assembling itself.

"We should look at hotels. The ones near the park." He set his cup down. His jaw shifted once, eyes moving left and back. "The one on the water. We looked at it before. The Inn."

"Bar Harbor Inn."

“Bar Harbor.” He said it with the small release of a man who had found what he was looking for — though he hadn't found it. I handed it to him without thinking, the way you hand someone something they've dropped, the exchange too small to require acknowledgment.

“Your shoulder,” Paul said.

“It’s alright.”

“Better than yesterday?”

“Yeah. How are you doing?”

He looked at his hands on the table. He had developed the habit of watching them the way I had developed the habit of watching his face — not constantly, not obviously, but with the low peripheral attention of someone running a continuous check.

“I got stuck this morning,” he said.

“What?”

“Not with moving. Stuck on a thought. Before you came down. I was going to make a list. Things to do before Acadia.”

“How long?”

“Ten minutes. Maybe more.” His thumb moved along the handle of his cup. “I could see the items. I knew exactly what the list needed.”

“I guess seeing the thing is not the same as naming it.”

“No,” he said. “It isn't.”

“The list gets made,” I said. “Just later.”

His right one kept a fine, steady rhythm. *He’s not hiding it anymore.*

“I finished it before I came to get you.” He smiled. “Eleven items.”

He said, "Actually, twelve. I added binoculars."

"Binoculars?"

"You can't go to Acadia without binoculars. There are birds."

"I know there are birds."

His chin lifted a fraction, the way he might if he was listening to something. A chair scraped. The two men near the window began putting on their coats. Paul picked up his coffee, took a sip, and set it down.

Outside, a woman walked past with a child who moved at the stop-start pace of someone for whom the world was full of things worth stopping for. The woman's hand was loose around the child's — not pulling, not restraining, just present.

"The binoculars are in the hall closet," I said. "Top shelf."

"I know where they are."

"You put them on the list."

"As a reminder," he said, with the dignity of a man who held his position under pressure.

I laughed, "For next year." He looked at me the way he had looked at me across kitchen tables for twenty years — patient, a little amused, entirely himself.

He nodded toward my cup. "It's getting cold."

I drank my tea. The coffee shop moved at the speed of the world — conversations quick and fluid, thoughts arriving and departing.

"Next September," Paul said.

"About thirteen months," I said. *We are still going to do this.* I sipped my tea. *This is living.*

CHAPTER 58

Tuesday, September 15

It started with Gerald, the way things in room 107 often started — sideways, disguised as something else, arriving before anyone had agreed to let it in.

Gerald was looking at his phone. "Can I ask something that might sound stupid?"

"Gerald," Linda said, "you have never asked anything stupid."

He set the phone face-down on his knee. "When the doctor tells you it's the dopamine cells, it's the basal ganglia, it's the substantia nigra — when they give you all the geography of it." He paused, looking at his hands. "Does anyone else feel like that's not quite right? Like the map isn't the place?"

"Say more," Linda said.

"I know my brain is different. I know my chemistry has changed." He turned his hands over. "But when I'm sitting here talking to you — when I'm in this room, when I'm still annoyed about the coffee, or I look at Diane's whatever-that-is—"

"It's a hat," Diane said without looking up.

"When I look at Diane's hat," Gerald said, "I feel like myself. Not a damaged version of myself. Just me." He paused. "So, which is it? Am I my brain chemistry? Or am I simply — me?"

"That is the question," Tara said.

Dr. Patel leaned forward slightly. "In medicine, we treat the brain. The body. That's what we have tools for." She paused. "But you're asking about something the tools don't reach."

She looked at Gerald, then Linda. "Consciousness researchers have been trying to answer this for decades — what is the relationship between the brain and the experience of being you? They call it the hard problem. It's hard because you can map everything the brain does and still not explain why there is an inside to any of it."

Gerald said, "Inside of what?"

Dr. Patel said, "How you are you."

Gerald nodded.

"The subjective experience," Tara said. She looked around the circle. "No one knows where your awareness comes from. Whether it's produced by the brain or expressed through it."

"Through it?" Martin said. "Like we aren't in our heads?"

"Some researchers think the self is more like a field than a location," Tara said. "Not housed in any set of cells. Not necessarily in the head, or the body, or anywhere fixed."

"Like a soul," I said. "Who we are — we persist."

Tara looked at me and nodded.

A week earlier, Paul had been reading at the kitchen table. He'd looked up mid-page and read aloud without preamble — the way he did when something struck him as too important to wait. "The evidence suggests that consciousness is expressed through the neural systems, not produced by them." Paul lowered the book and said, "That tells me consciousness can't arise from our neurons. If it did, as our neurons died, parts of who we are would die with them."

I had lain awake that night turning the idea over. I thought about the episode, when I'd gone too long without levodopa — the way the world became slow and strange. Even though my body stopped working, I was still there. Behind it. Watching.

The next morning, Paul had come downstairs dressed in his Sunday clothes and said, "I'm going to church. Want to come?"

Dr. Patel's description of consciousness connected to something on the edge of my understanding. I said to the room, "Maybe who we are isn't an extinguishable flame. Maybe we are more."

"Yes," Gerald said. "That."

"Is that what you mean?" Linda asked him. "When you say you feel like yourself — is that it?"

Gerald nodded slowly. "I've lost things. Parkinson's likes to steal everything. But I haven't gone anywhere."

Diane set down her knitting. "I keep expecting Parkinson's to learn it can't erase me." She paused. "Slow learner."

Several people laughed.

Michelle said, "If you persist — can you survive even the worst of Parkinson's?" She hesitated. "Or does dementia take you in a way Parkinson's can't?"

I thought about Mrs. Henderson in the memory care unit. *What is it like to be her...knowing she is being erased?*

Then I thought about Eleanor, waiting in my laptop. Eleanor had understood things I hadn't...things about myself…only discovered after I wrote the words, as if I'd known all along.

"I've been writing a novel," I said.

The room looked at me. Rebecca smiled.

"My character," I said. "Eleanor. She understood things I couldn't have told you consciously. But they were in me. I wrote them."

"Yes," Tara said.

Sarah was holding Tom's hand. He was looking out of the window. "Knowing this," she said quietly, "knowing that Parkinson's...maybe even dementia...doesn't take who you are. What do we do with that?"

CHAPTER 59

Tuesday, September 15

Gerald said, "Tara, you've been listening to all of us. You've said a few things." He paused. He looked at her steadily. "You're a doctor. You treat this disease. And now you have it." He paused. "What's that like?"

Tara looked at Gerald for a long moment.

"I believed," she said, "that understanding the aging process would make it different when time came for me."

"Then I didn't just age...Parkinson's. I know what the data says." She paused. "I believed — I think I genuinely believed — that being a neurologist would create some distance between me and the thing itself. That knowledge would function as a buffer." She stopped.

She started again. "It doesn't. There is no distance. Knowing makes it slower in some ways. In other ways it makes it—"

She said, “More detailed. I know exactly what is happening. I know the name of every symptom before it arrives.” She took a deep breath. “Knowing the name of a thing is not the same as being prepared for it.”

She touched her forehead.

“I'm a neurologist. I knew what the symptoms were. But when I experienced them, I explained them away, anyway. For almost a year.” She looked up. “February was when I ran out of other explanations.”

She said, “I gave a new patient the diagnosis eight weeks ago,” She shook her head. “I've watched that moment many times. I've always believed I was giving people something real in those appointments — not just information, but presence. Care.”

Gerald said, “And now?”

“I understand that my patients and I are the same. I don't know whether the doctor’s desk or years of training helped her or me. I've been trying to figure that out and I can't quite get there.”

CHAPTER 60

Friday, October 2

I heard Paul walking down the hall before I was fully awake. He started the morning ritual. I lay there and listened. The routine stopped, replaced by silence. The silence continued.

I got up.

He was standing at the counter, facing the window, the blue cup in his hand, coffee poured, nothing wrong. The light coming through the glass was pale. Paul was simply standing there, cup in hand, not drinking.

I watched him from the doorway before coming in. I got my cup, poured my coffee and stood beside him at the counter.

Paul said, “I was trying to remember.”

I waited.

"The tremor." He looked at his hand on the cup. "There must have been a last morning when I didn't think about it. When I just — made the coffee." He paused. "I can't find it. I keep going back and I can't find the last ordinary morning."

I didn't look at his face. I looked out the window and breathed in through my nose, slowly, the way I had learned to breathe when something needed to be carried rather than put down.

"I did the math again last night," he said. "After you were asleep."

"I know."

He looked at me.

"You had your phone under the covers," I said. "You think I can't tell."

"The progression models—"

"Are models."

"Joy."

"They are averages. Populations. They are not you standing in this kitchen."

He was quiet.

"I know," he said. "I know that when I'm thinking correctly." He set the cup down. "And then it's three in the morning."

I had been where he was standing. Not this kitchen, not three in the morning with his phone under the covers, but that same place — the one where the ground you thought was solid reveals itself as something you had simply never tested. I had stood there alone because he had not known the place and I had not known how to bring him in. I had found my way through and come out on the other side into something that was not exactly acceptance but was at least a place where you could make coffee and drink it.

He was at the entrance to all of that now, and I was the only person in the room who knew what was on the other side, and I could not carry him through it.

"The mornings get ordinary again," I said. "Not the same ordinary. A different one."

He looked at me with the look of a man who needed that to be true and was not yet sure it was.

"It takes time," I said. "And then one morning you're just standing here and you're not doing the math."

"How long?"

I thought of a number. The kindness of a number, even an invented one. I thought about him at three in the morning, running the models, looking for the variable that changed the outcome.

"I don't know," I said.

We stood at the counter while the sun's light strengthened without warming. The dew was still on the grass. A mockingbird started up somewhere in the neighbor's yard and then stopped, as though it had reconsidered.

After a while, Paul said, "I should look up the sparrows."

"What?"

"The ones in the back hedge. I keep meaning to identify them." He looked out the window.

"They're sparrows."

He said, "I've been assuming they're song sparrows, but the markings aren't quite right."

"How long have you been looking at them?"

"Three weeks," he said, with the composure of a man who had been conducting a private investigation and was only now disclosing it. "I've been watching from the kitchen window. I'd need the binoculars to be sure."

I looked at the hedge, the small movements in it, the birds I had stopped seeing because they were always there.

"Get the binoculars," I said.

He set his cup down and went to find them, his bare feet hardly heard as he walked across the kitchen. It was a relief, an ordinary sound of a man moving through his home on a morning that had returned, for the moment, to just being a morning.

CHAPTER 61

Tuesday, October 20

"I want to go somewhere different," Linda said. "Death."

She let the word settle before continuing. "What have you told your family? Has anyone made advance directives? Are you afraid of thinking about dying?" She looked around the circle. "Who wants to start?"

Robert said, "I've done the paperwork. DNR. Healthcare proxy. All of it." He looked at his cane across his knees. "My wife cried. My son said I was being morbid. My daughter said it was sensible."

Diane said, "I've been thinking about this for a while. It's not morbid. It's mine to think about. It's the one thing in this whole business I still get to decide."

"It's not the dying that bothers me," Robert said. "Not particularly. I'm afraid of the part before. The part where I'm present but not reachable. Where my wife is in the room and I can see her." He gestured with his hand, raising it with emphasis. "I want to still be findable when she looks for me. That's what I want. I know I might not get it." He looked out of the window. "But that's what I want."

I thought about Paul Friday morning at the counter, cup in hand, the coffee going cold while he stood in the full weight of what he knew was coming. He had been entirely there — that was the thing nobody told you, that the hardest moments were not the ones where the disease took you somewhere else but the ones where you stayed completely present inside your own fear.

"I haven't done the paperwork," Owen said. "Two months in, I don't think I need to worry about it. I mean, if I do the paperwork or even think like that, I'm admitting this is the direction. I guess I believe that by avoiding thinking like that...well, it means the direction is still undecided. Maybe I can outrun Parkinson's. Maybe I won't get dementia." He looked up. "I know that's not how it works."

"No," Gerald said. "It's not. But two months in, you're allowed to not have done it yet. But I suppose we're all doomed, soon as we're born. Might as well get used to the idea."

Owen replied, "When did you?"

Gerald said, "After I named the shower chair. Different thresholds." He picked up his coffee and made the face that had become the room's reliable dark joke. He made the face, despite the coffee's improvement.

Paul said, "Some of us need more data points, before we can think about it."

Jennifer had been fidgeting. "I did it a couple months ago. Not because I was ready. Because I needed to feel like I had done something practical." She paused. "It didn't make the idea of dying smaller. But it gave it a place to go. But seriously, Parkinson's isn't likely to kill any of us...at least not any time soon."

Across the circle, Tara sat with her hands open in her lap. I imagined her guiding such conversations — phrasing the questions, managing the pacing. But she said nothing.

Michelle said quietly that she hadn't told her extended family that she had Parkinson's. "I'm not ready to say it. I don't know when I will be. It's a decision I will make, eventually, I guess. Maybe this...death...is like that."

"The deciding is harder than telling," Linda said. "Once you've told them it's done."

"Alright, let's move on to something more hopeful. Experimental treatments. Like stem cell therapy." Linda said. "Who's looking at options?"

Owen looked up with the alertness of someone who had been waiting for this.

"I found three trials I'm eligible for," he said. "I've talked to my neurologist." He glanced at Tara and then away — the reflex of a patient who had just remembered he was looking at his doctor. "I'm going to enroll in one of them." He paused. "I know the success rates. I know the risk profile. I'm still going. I need to be doing something with this besides sitting with it."

"There's a trial using acupuncture points," Rebecca said. "The safety data is solid." She paused. "I'm not giving you medical advice. I'm saying that the research is worth reading."

"Have you considered anything?" Owen asked her.

"I've looked carefully," Rebecca said. "I'm thinking of getting a vibration plate, to help with balance, and maybe a red-light panel." She paused. "Other than that, I've decided to stick with what's working right now and reassess how things are going in six months. By then, I'm hoping the trial I'm waiting for will start."

Paul said, "What's the trial?"

"It does the opposite of levodopa. It uses a repurposed drug to reduce dopamine build-up. But I'll decide later, after the animal models are completed. So, for now I'm using a few supplements and exercise."

Paul's mouth dropped open. He looked at me before speaking. "That doesn't make sense. Why reduce dopamine? Isn't that the problem?"

"I know it sounds wrong. But I've done a lot of reading in medical journals. It would take a while to explain my reasoning. But it makes sense...at least to me it does. It's not a verdict on how anyone else should go forward."

Gerald said, "The people who do best, in my experience — not medical experience, just spending time in this room — are the ones who decide based on what they know, in their own bodies, rather than making decisions based on what we're supposed to do." He looked at Paul. Something silent exchanged between them.

Paul said, "I think you're right. I've been performing stability, predictability, following the rules, if there are rules for how to live with Parkinson's."

"The question of when presence becomes performance," Linda said. "That's one of the most honest things that comes up in this room."

"What if you can't notice" Owen asked, "the difference between performing and presence?"

"You keep coming back until you can," Diane said, without looking up. "That's what next week is for. And the next. And the next."

"The trying to notice is the thing," Gerald said. He looked at Diane, who was nodding at him. "Paul, for what it's worth — what you said before. Some of it was probably performance. But I think a lot of what you were doing was real."

Rebecca said, "Rock Steady Boxing. It's exercise for people with Parkinson's. There's a class twice a week. I just started." She glanced over at Gerald and smiled. "I think of it as working toward taking back myself."

CHAPTER 62

Thursday, October 22

The neighbor's' wind chimes found the breeze before we reached the porch steps — the long aluminum tubes hanging from strings on the oak, never quite in tune with anything. The sound arrived and dissolved and arrived again the way it had for years, without ever resolving into something you could accept or argue with.

I will never make peace with those chimes.

Paul took the chair closest to the door. I took the other one. We sat without talking for a while and then without a word of decision, we stood up and began to walk.

The walk would take about forty minutes. Two miles through the neighborhood. The leaves were coming down, inviting us to think about New England in the fall. We spoke about Acadia and the trail Paul had read about.

He said, "It runs along the cliffs above the ocean."

We had not talked about what he had said at Tuesday's meeting. I walked around it, the way I might walk around quicksand, knowing the danger.

Back on the porch, we sat once again in our assigned chairs.

"I've been thinking. He turned his hands over on the armrests. He looked as though he was trying to understand something from a distance. "Every time I think about a structured program — an exercise class — it stops being a thing I want to do and becomes a thing I'm supposed to do." He paused. "And then I don't do it."

I looked at the neighbor's oak tree with its chimes. Then I shifted to look across the street. Mrs. Henderson's chimes were as silent as her house, now left empty and waiting.

"The walk tonight wasn't medicine," I said.

"No."

"But it was."

"Yes," he said. "But it didn't feel like it while we were doing it."

The wind chimes lifted and fell. Three notes that didn't resolve. *There's something missing in the sound.*

"I've been going to the gym," Paul said.

"Really?"

"Three times a week since September. I don't tell anyone there about the Parkinson's." He paused. "Nobody knows my name. Nobody asks questions. Nobody watches my form to see if the disease is showing." He looked at the street. "It's where I'm just a man at a gym."

"So ... that's where you've been going. I was wondering. Why didn't you tell me?"

He was quiet for a moment. "Because telling you would make it a Parkinson's thing," he said. "And I needed it to not be a Parkinson's thing. I needed one place where I was just going." He paused. "I know that doesn't entirely make sense."

"It makes complete sense," I said.

A woman with a stroller passed on the sidewalk, her pace even, the baby's hand visible over the edge reaching at the darkening air.

"The trail will be like that," Paul said.

"How so?"

"A gym is neutral. I have no history with it."

History. Yes. That's the sound that's missing. The clunk of Mrs. Henderson's broken wind chime.

"We know this neighborhood," Paul said. "We have a version of us here. There, we'll be different."

"I think I get what you're saying" I said.

Paul said, "I'm tired of grieving."

"I think the grieving and acceptance happen at the same time. Neither one waits for the other to finish." I looked at the street. "But a hiking trail is still a trail. A river still sounds the same before you see it. And our neighborhood, it's still what it is. We're the ones working through stuff."

A car passed, its headlights swept across us.

"Is that what you did?" he said. "Just said, life is what it is?"

"I'm still finding my way. Every day is different."

The wind chimes moved again. T*hat is exactly what our life has become. Not living. Not a solvable problem. I live inside of an irritating sound.*

"I hate those chimes," I said.

"They're not going anywhere."

"No," I said. "They're not."

I could tell he knew I wasn't talking about the chimes.

CHAPTER 63

Thursday, October 22

Paul said, "If you invest in something and it doesn't work — if you do everything right and the disease does what it does anyway — the hoping makes it worse than if you hadn't hoped at all."

"After the diagnosis, I read everything I could," I said. "And then one morning I woke up and understood that the research had become...Oh, how do I say it? ... For me, research was my nightlight. I didn't just use it to see. It made the dark feel smaller."

He said, "I remember. It was like you were obsessed with knowing as much as your doctor."

"I think it was important for me to do that. Reading medical journals was doing something. It was a way to say, No."

Paul squeezed my hand.

"I think hoping is the same," I said. "You hope carefully. You don't commit to it. You hold it at a distance so if it doesn't work, you can say you never fully believed it would." I looked at the street. "I've been doing that with Dr. Patel's card."

"Do you mean the message about Rock Steady or trusting yourself?"

"Both."

"Why?" Paul swatted at a bug.

"If I walk into Rock Steady," I said, "I will see someone further along than me. I know this. I know that is what I will see — someone whose hands I recognize from somewhere ahead on the road I'm on. And I will understand, standing there in a boxing class, exactly where I'm headed." I paused. "As long as I don't go, I don't have to see that."

"But you see it every Tuesday."

That's different. We're just sitting, talking, thinking. There, people are hoping, trying, fighting. And if I see it doesn't work…if people are still progressing…in a program meant to slow the progression…then what hope is there?"

"And there's the other thing," Paul said. "Rock Steady is what you do instead of the thing you used to do. It's the Parkinson's version of the thing that was just yours."

"I think," he said slowly, "that we're both protecting something that doesn't exist anymore."

CHAPTER 64

Thursday, October 22

It was dark but neither of us moved to go inside.

"There's something else," Paul said. "About the gym."

I leaned back in my chair.

Paul said, "Some days I get to the parking lot and I sit there," he said. "Engine off. I know what I'm there for." He paused. "And I sit there for ten minutes because something between knowing what I'm there for and actually getting out of the car has gone quiet."

He said, "I used to just get out of the car. I've been getting out of cars my entire life without thinking about it." He paused. "Now, some days there's this gap...between the intention and the beginning. I sit in that gap, and I wait for it to close and eventually it closes and I get out."

"Yeah. I can relate."

"But I don't know if it's going to close every time. I don't know if one day it just — doesn't."

"That's probably because you're getting old." I laughed.

Paul laughed as he said, "I am not."

"Seriously. I think it might be a symptom," I said. "That's not weakness. I mean, I haven't given up. But then everything feels flat."

"Flat? That's a good way to put it. Does it help to know that?" he asked. "That it's neurological."

"It helps with the self-blame," I said. "It doesn't help with getting out of the car."

He made a sound that was almost a laugh. "No," he said. "I suppose it doesn't."

"I asked Rebecca about that. How she goes to Rock Steady even when she doesn't feel the motivation or the energy to go. What helps with getting out of the car?"

"And?"

"She said it was easier each time. Doing it once makes the next time slightly smaller. And the time after that, easier again."

Paul said, "Like she accumulated evidence?"

"What do you mean?"

"Proof. That she could do the class. Kept going until her body started to trust what she was doing."

We sat together, the evening disturbed by the wind chimes.

"I've been thinking about what it would feel like," I said. "Walking into Rock Steady. Not what I'm afraid of; I've thought about that enough. What it might feel like." I paused. "Rebecca said people move like they mean it."

I turned in the chair to look at Paul directly. "I don't know when I started making myself smaller. I don't think I noticed while it was happening. You just stop doing one thing, and then another, and then another, and one day you look up and the life you're living is the size of the things you haven't stopped doing yet."

"Like not seeing your friends anymore?" Paul said.

"Yeah. And not going to celebrations or bowling. Bit by bit, I've laid things down."

"That's your book," he said. "What you just said. That's Eleanor."

"Maybe I'll go," I said.

Paul was quiet.

"Not a commitment," I said. "A maybe. I'm saying there is a version of life in which I pick up that card and call the number of Rock Steady."

CHAPTER 65

Monday, November 2

Paul held my door open. Then he got in and sat without starting the engine. The quiet between us had the texture of two people who had been somewhere together and had said things there that were still settling. Not the quiet of the drive over — that had been two people preparing. These were two people who had been inside something and were not yet ready to leave it.

"I'm still afraid," he said.

"I know."

"The data is real. The risk of discontinuation is real."

"I know it is. But Dr. Patel is helping me. I'm weaning off levodopa. Not just stopping."

"I don't know," he said.

"You don't have to stop using it," I said. "This is something I want to do. For me."

"I know." He put the key into the ignition. "Would we rather decline together or one at a time?"

He had asked this before. In the kitchen, months ago, when the question was still theoretical.

"Together," I said. "But I don't want the managed version of us any more than I want the managed version of me."

"Together," he said. "Alright. I'll try not to complain about your choice. So long as you follow Doctor Patel's instructions on how to stop using the levodopa. I don't agree. But I understand."

CHAPTER 66

Saturday, November 14

Our street in the morning was unhurried, a little loose at the edges, with the weather still deciding what kind of day it was going to be. I had taken to walking differently...not wholly a compensation but an adjustment.

The physical therapist had shown me how to think about heel strike, to look at a visual target ahead. He gave me a full routine of calf stretching — first one way and then the other — all in hopes of eliminating footdrop.

Though scuffing my toes now and again was a minor issue, Dr. Patel pointed out that it could develop into a serious fall. Dr Patel said, "And swing your arms. It may feel weird. Like you're exaggerating the swing. That's what you want. Buildup, until you can do big arm swings while walking fast."

So, I was walking by myself, which left me with an abundance of thinking time.

The thing you have left, after the thing you were is gone, is yourself. Just yourself, without the role.

I had been thinking about that since Tuesday. Not the way I used to think about things — filing them, managing them, taking them home and placing them carefully in a category and closing the drawer. Just thinking. Letting the thought move around in me and seeing where it went.

I was in the middle of a profound thought when I found the thing lying on the ground, near the base of Henderson's fence. It was half hidden under a pile of wet leaves that the wind had gathered against the fence post. I knew it was Mrs. Henderson's wind chime, the one that was broken and offered only a sad clunking sound. Someone had taken it down, or the wind had, or it had simply given up hope after years of weather and neglect and a house that no longer had anyone in it paying attention to what it had to say.

I considered picking it up. I had no idea why I should and even argued with myself about bending over for the thing. *I hate wind chimes. Maybe that's as good a reason as any to pick the thing up.*

Holding it up, the hollow tubes made a faint knocking sound when the wind moved them, showing that, even though it was broken, the chime struggled to live. A small maple leaf was caught in the strings. The leaf was dried out and amber colored even its edges. I didn't remove it. The leaf had arrived there by its own means, and it was now part of what the wind chime was.

CHAPTER 67

Saturday, November 14

I set the wind chime on the kitchen counter. "Mrs. Henderson's," I said.

Paul looked at it for a moment. He touched its bent tubes and cracked disc. Paul pointed at the small amber leaf caught in the strings. I smiled.

I found the hammer and a nail and hung the chime on the wall beside the back door. Not outside, where the wind would move it. The absence of ringing or clunking was, at least in part, the point. Inside, it was frozen on the wall. I would see it every time I went out and again when I returned. The chime would be what it was — broken but still here, with an amber leaf caught in its strings for as long as the leaf lasted.

I stepped back and looked at it. *Perfect. That is what staying looks like from the inside.*

CHAPTER 68

Wednesday, November 18

Staying present was the thing I kept returning to, sitting across from Paul in the living room with the dark pressing against the windows. It had not been a bad day in any way I could point to.

Nothing had happened. Nothing had fallen or been dropped or lost. The medications had been on time. Paul was taking his usual dose. Dr. Patel had been reducing my medication. I was down to half a pill, taken only in the morning.

Paul and I cooked dinner together and cleaned up afterwards...together. Really, it was a decent day.

It had simply worn me out.

Paul was in his chair. The lamp beside him was on, which meant he had intended to read, but the book was closed on his knee and had been closed for an hour. His right hand rested on top of it, the tremor doing its work.

He was looking at the middle distance, the way he looked at it in the evenings when the levodopa had finished its arc. He had taken a pill a few minutes ago and was waiting for the "on" to start. I could see where Paul was — just there — in the nowhere of a body that had spent its available resources and was waiting to be replenished.

I knew the place of his look. I had not seen this look on Paul before October. Now I could identify it from across the room. I could tell it from ordinary tiredness. I could read the difference between Paul resting and Paul depleted. On and off. I was becoming fluent in a language I had never wanted to learn and could not unlearn...the language of caregiving.

I was running on what remained of my last dose and there was no levodopa coming to my rescue.

I should say something.

There is nothing worth the effort to say.

I had words. I knew how to fill a room with language when language was what the room needed. I had been doing it for months...using words to steady Paul. It required careful work to stay present, to be available just in case questions were asked, grief grew too heavy, or something was forgotten. The reward had been long lazy evenings threaded through with conversation and touch.

But tonight, there was nothing in me.

The fluctuation in energy and motivation, it's a part of Parkinson's rarely spoken about. Dr. Patel had warned me about it, while explaining how we would reduce my medication. "No levodopa may mean no energy. More apathy. Increased symptoms. But the dip in energy, you might feel that the most."

I wanted to talk to Paul. But what really can be said, when you reach empty at the same time your husband is starting to perk back up?

"Are you alright?" he said. Not a question, exactly. More like: I see you. I want to ask. But I'm asking from a very great distance.

"No," I said. "Are you?"

"Getting there," he said.

We sat with that.

He reached for something to say — I could see it happen. He found nothing…or said nothing, which I supposed was the same thing. So, we sat there, Paul waking up with the help of the medicine and me drifting without it.

"I hate this," Paul said.

"Me too," I said.

That was all that was worthwhile to say, because it was the only true thing to say now.

The simplest possible acknowledgment of the simplest possible truth, which was that we were both here.

I got up.

Paul watched me. There was a question in his look — not alarm, just attention.

"I need a few minutes," I said.

His nod was not an agreement to my choice to stop taking levodopa. The nod said: I know. Go. Come back.

I went to the kitchen.

I didn't turn on the light. I stood in the dark kitchen with the world continuing outside the window...just stood there and didn't do anything.

In the other room, Paul's lamp was still on. I could see the edge of its light from where I stood.

Somehow, I'd lost the expectation that his light would come on whenever I needed him. I didn't need to say "I am fine" when I wasn't. I was just happy knowing that his lamp was still on. Paul was still there, waiting in the living room, reading his book or maybe just sitting there, looking at nothing. And I stayed in the dark kitchen a little longer.

CHAPTER 69

Saturday, December 5

Paul appeared in the kitchen with his coat on and the question in his expression rather than in his words. It was cold out — winter had arrived without the drama of northern winters but settled in the bones anyway. His coat had become a kind of shorthand between us that asked, *ready for our walk?*

The park was a municipal thing — a paved loop around a modest pond, some benches, and trees that were bare. We had been walking the loop since November. Once a week, sometimes twice. The path was flat enough and the surface was reliable. There was a bench at the end of the pond where we sometimes stopped.

We sat on the bench.

The heron is gone. I noted its absence saying, "Smart birds follow the warmth. Do you think Mr. Heron was smart?"

Paul said, "Possibly. Or maybe it just went somewhere else."

"The pond looks lower."

Paul had been quiet for most of the walk.

"I've been reading more," he said.

"You're always reading."

"About Oregon. About the other states."

"How many now?"

He didn't answer right off and then said, "That's not important."

I looked at the far bank, where a stand of bare sycamores stood, taking a spotlight against the gray of winter.

"I've been reading the arguments against," he said. "Not just the ones I expected."

"Like?"

"The disability rights people." He paused. "Not the religious argument. I understand the religious argument — I don't share it, but I understand it. The disability rights argument is different. It unsettles me more."

We'd had this talk before, and it had left me disturbed. I thought that perhaps Paul had set it aside. I was not happy to learn that he had not.

He pulled his coat tighter. "The concern is that when you make assisted death legal — when you build the structure and the system and the safeguards — you also, unavoidably, build a message into the culture."

I waited for him to continue, but he seemed lost in his own thoughts. "What message?"

“That some lives are worth ending. That suffering past a certain point requires a reasonable off-ramp. And the people who are already living those lives — the people for whom others already find it difficult to imagine their quality of life — they feel that message. They feel it in how they're treated. In how doctors speak to them. In the assumptions made about what they must want."

I sat with that, watching a squirrel scampering, hunting for his lost nuts, most likely.

"I hadn't thought about it like that. Truth is, I haven’t given it much thought," I said.

"I hadn't either. I thought the argument was going to be the slippery slope — the expansion of criteria over time, which is also real. That troubles me. But this was something else. The idea that the option itself changes the culture around disability and dying. Around what counts as a life worth living."

“How would it affect us. I mean, we’re not suffering. So, why think about it?”

Paul said, “There are people who have neurodegeneration that go to a doctor for something else. Like say, cancer or heart disease. And someone, the system let’s say, decides they don’t need treatment because what’s the point of spending money on old people, or people who already have a brain issue.”

I said, “Save the money and resources for those who are younger, who don’t have a neurological problem?”

“That’s the concern. And there is some evidence that this is already starting. There are cases of individuals who have down syndrome, MS, dementia, or Parkinson’s.”

“And?”

“They are denied care. It’s illegal. But by the time something is done to fix the issue, sue an insurance company, force compliance, people have died.”

"But then," I said, "the other side of that —"

Paul nodded.

"The person trapped in a bed or inside their body," I said.

"Yes." He tossed a stone at the water. It fell short, landing on the bank.

A dog appeared on the path behind us — an old lab, moving slowly. It looked at us with the mild interest of an animal for whom most things had become familiar, and then it moved on.

"What troubles me," I said, after a while, "is the question of coercion. Not the obvious kind. Not someone leaning over a bed saying *you should.* The quiet kind. The feeling — whether it comes from inside or outside, whether it's real or imagined — that you are a burden. That the people who love you are exhausted. That the reasonable thing, the considerate thing, would be to leave life."

"Yes."

"How do you make that choice freely," I said, "when you're living inside that much dependence. When you can feel what it costs."

"I've thought about that from the other direction," he said. "From where I stand. Whether I want the door — or is it about autonomy. Or not wanting death to cost too much, not financially, I mean physically, emotionally.”

"I don't know," I said.

"I think there's something in the choosing that's genuinely mine. The sense that I want to be the one who decides, not a disease. That feels real." He paused. "But I can't rule out my other concern. You. About not wanting you to mourn. And I also don't want you taking care of me, if I don't remember you."

"I'll remind you if you forget."

The owner of the lab appeared around the bend, a woman in her seventies, unhurried, a wool hat low over her ears. She raised her hand as she passed. We waved back.

I said, "The religious argument — the one you said you understand but don't share."

"Yes."

"I keep coming back to it sideways. Not the doctrine. But the thing underneath it — the idea that suffering might be — not good, not something to seek — but not only loss. That something good can happen in suffering. That there's a version of the end of a life that is also a kind of — completion. That witnessing one's own death might matter."

He looked at me. "You think that? And I thought I was being morbid."

"I don't know what I think," I said. "I hold it the same way you hold the disability argument. It unsettles me. I don't want to romanticize suffering. But I also don't want to...I don't want to decide in advance that there's nothing in the hard part. Like deciding God screwed up by making the possibility of suffering. That I know better than God and can make the best or the rational choice. Sanitize life and then exit cleanly."

"And yet."

"You want the door," I said. "I get it. I think I want it to exist. I just — I'm not sure I trust my ability to know, from this side, what I would decide."

"Probably no one can know," Paul adjusted his hat. "Maybe the right to die is kind of not applicable to most people. I mean, most people who want to leave, don't need a law saying they can do it."

I laughed. "Right. Are they going to put a corpse in prison?"

"Joy. Sometimes I worry about you."

"Me? I didn't bring up the topic."

"If it were available here, in Arkansas," he said. "Would you?"

I held the question, twisting the hem of my coat sleeve. "I don't know."

"I'm the same," he said.

"What I keep coming back to," he said, "is that the conversation we're having — the fact that we can have it, that we're having it now, clearly, while we still can — this is what I wanted." He looked back at the water. "Whatever we decide. I wanted us to have said it while we could still say it clearly."

A bird landed not ten feet from us, moved, looked at us briefly, and flew away.

The exit door is there. I hope neither of us ever needs to decide.

We got up from the bench and walked.

CHAPTER 70

Sunday, December 6

I found her in the garage. Not her, exactly. The box was labeled in my handwriting: Mom — music. I had written that with a Sharpie at her kitchen table two weeks after the funeral, when my sister and I divided what remained between us, and I was not yet in a condition to make real decisions. The music box included everything I could not categorize.

I was looking for a flashlight. Paul had asked me to check the garage because the power had flickered twice that morning. Paul was the kind of man who needed a working flashlight the moment the power flickered, even if the sun was up and there were eleven candles in the drawer. I did not find the flashlight. But I found the box.

The flashlight is probably in the drawer too.

I set the box on the workbench.

The tape had yellowed and stiffened. It lifted when I put my fingers under it; the adhesive had gone soft with time. I opened the flaps.

A paperback, spine broken, pages fanned — *Selected Poems of Emily Dickinson.* My mother's copy. Her handwriting in the margins, small and tilted slightly right, was the handwriting of a woman who had formed opinions and wanted a record of when she'd formed them. I opened it to an annotated page. "I'm Nobody! Who are you?" The margin notes beside it read: "Students always laugh at this one because they think she's being cute."

Underneath the book was a stack of greeting cards. The rubber band holding them together was brittle, breaking when I tried to remove it. Cards she had saved, curled from time — birthdays, a few Christmas cards, several with no occasion at all. I had sent her some of them

My handwriting in my twenties was rounder, more confident. It was the handwriting of a person who had not yet learned to worry about handwriting. On a postcard from Vermont, I had written, "Just thinking about you."

She kept it.

There were photographs. Not the ones a person would choose to put in a photo album. Those had gone to my sister. These were the loose ones, undated, the ones my mother had not gotten around to putting anywhere.

My parents on a beach I didn't recognize. They still looked young. It felt as if I were looking at strangers who bore a resemblance to people I knew.

My sister and I, ages six and four, were on some porch, squinting at whoever was holding the camera.

My mother at her classroom desk, stacks of papers on each side of her, looking up at something outside the frame with the expression of a woman in the middle of something that interested her.

I set the photograph on the workbench.

I had not looked at her face for a long time. I had been carrying a composite in my head — her voice, the vocabulary of her opinions, the way she could hold an argument open and examine it before deciding which side she was on. The face in the photograph was younger than she was in my memory, sharper. It was the face of a person who had not yet been ill.

She would have been seventy-two in November. She would have known what to say.

I kept the bad memory at a distance, the way I kept other things at a distance. I put it on the shelf I had told Paul about, after the episode. I said, "Dark thoughts don't go anywhere. Dark jokes are avoidance. If I want to live, I need to break the contract I've made. Reclaim who I used to be." Paul smiled and said he thought that was a good idea...said he had missed me.

But the work of reclamation wasn't going very well. Fact was, I had doubts. *Is my intention possible? Is it what I really want?*

My mother had believed, with the conviction of a woman who taught Dickinson and Chekhov and *The Bluest Eye* for three decades, that "the right words spoken into the right silence became a door." What happened next was between the words and the person who heard them. She said, "It's important to hold the door open."

That was the thing I could honestly say to myself, standing in the garage with her photograph on the workbench and Emily Dickinson in my hands. I hadn't taken her approach to life. Instead of opening doors, I had been closing them.

My mother would have recognized this as existing in what she called, "failure mode."

When I was thirty-two and my parents were divorcing, I refused to talk to either of them about what was happening. I said, "Whatever you two decide is fine. It's not my life. So, whatever."

Mother had looked at me and said, "Joy. You know what Dickinson said about telling the truth."

"Tell all the truth but tell it slant." I said, because she had made me memorize it.

"Not a lie," she said. "Straight. Just take the long way around if you must, so it doesn't blind anyone. But tell it. Tell all of it."

I've taken the long way around life, to the point that slanting has feathered into a lie.

Mrs. Henderson said that going is the point. Not what I managed to do when I was there. Just the going.

My mother knew this...had been trying to tell me something like it, through Dickinson.

The flashlight was in the drawer, as I had suspected. I found it in thirty seconds and went back inside. Paul was sitting at the kitchen table.

"Found it," I said, setting the box on the floor.

"I knew you would. Everything all right?"

I set the flashlight on the table and sat down.

"I found a box of my mother's things. She kept a card I sent her." I said, reaching across the table to turn Paul's mug.

He looked at me; his head tilted in question.

"It was crooked," I said.

He looked at the mug. "Thank you."

"You're welcome."

CHAPTER 71

Sunday, December 6

I was putting mother's box back in the garage after looking through it with Paul.

On the low shelf beside the camping equipment, there was a manila folder I didn't recognize. Cream-colored, with no label. It had the look of something placed carefully rather than forgotten.

I took the folder off the shelf.

Inside: newspaper clippings, some of them photocopied, some cut directly from the page. A sheaf of printouts, municipal documents, the kind with reference numbers in the header and language that had been written by committees. Several pages of handwritten notes on yellow legal paper.

I sat down on a five-gallon bucket of paint and read.

The subject across all the contents was the municipal water system — specifically a stretch of aging infrastructure that ran beneath the older residential streets on the east side, the ones built before the current codes, including ours. An assessment recommended that the town replace the pipes.

The handwritten notes documented meetings, city council sessions and committee hearings, in which Mrs. Henderson had apparently spoken several times. Her notes were precise: dates, names of commissioners, the specific language of the motions she had pushed for and eventually gotten.

There were follow-up letters that she had written and received. A final clipping announced the completion of the infrastructure replacement project for the east residential district. It was deemed a huge success, mostly because the project was finished under budget. It had been a project that a commissioner was quoted as calling, "long overdue."

I was still sitting there when Paul opened the door. He looked at me and saw the folder on my knees.

"You found it," he said.

"It was on the shelf."

"I put it there." He came out and sat down on the step near me. He looked at the folder rather than at me. "Her daughter gave it to me when they were clearing the house. She said her mother had wanted you to have it."

He picked up a newspaper clipping. "Said her mother had talked about the neighbor across the street, who seemed to be having a hard time. She thought you should know."

"Know what, exactly?"

Paul put the clipping back in the open folder.

"That the water is safe. That was what Mrs. Henderson wanted you to know. That she had made sure of it." He paused. "She pushed the city to replace the old infrastructure on these streets. They finally did. I guess she wanted credit, basically." Something moved on his face — not quite a smile. "That's what the daughter said. She wanted someone to know she'd done it."

"Why didn't you give it to me?"

"You'd stopped asking about the water," he said. "You went through that period, when you were very focused on the water. The smell. Then you stopped. You seem to have set it down. I didn't want to pick it back up for you."

He said, "I thought if I gave you the folder, it would reopen the question. Whether the water had something to do with the Parkinson's. Whether there was a cause to find."

He shook his head. "You seemed better without the question."

"The water had nothing to do with the smell."

"No. That's — that's what the folder says. The infrastructure was replaced."

I looked at the last clipping.

Paul had decided I was better without the folder. That was a version of the thing we had been doing for each other — providing managed kindness, protective withholding, making decisions about what could be handled. I had done it to him. He had done it to me. We had both called it consideration, and it had been that and something else.

"I would have wanted to know," I said. "Not whether the water smelled. I would have wanted to know what she did." I held the folder and said, "The daughter gave this to you because Mrs. Henderson wanted me to have it. She wanted me to know what she'd done."

"You're right," he said. "That was wrong. I did a lot of things wrong. I thought it was right, but it wasn't. You're my wife, not a glass China doll."

"Mrs. Henderson tended things," I said. "That was what she said she wanted. To still be someone who tended things." I looked at the folder. "She was. Right up until she couldn't be."

CHAPTER 72

Monday, December 7

Paul was in the bedroom, but not yet asleep. I could hear the quality of his not-sleeping from where I stood: the small adjustments, the pillow moved and moved again; the body conducting its negotiations with the hour. He would sleep eventually.

I had gotten up because my shoulder wanted me to. Not pain, exactly. But I needed to walk or stretch or do something besides lying in bed. I had learned not to argue with my body. Arguing cost more than getting up.

Paul turned the nightlight on. He does that for me.

At the kitchen sink, I turned on the tap. Cold water came out first, the pipes giving up what they'd been holding, and then warmer. I put my hands under the stream of water the way I'd been putting my hands into water my whole life without thinking about it.

The water ran over my hands. *Water receives whatever I put into it, moves around it and continues.* The water was warm now. I turned it a little cooler, the way I liked it. After I was satisfied with the result, I turned off the tap.

I dried my hands on the dish towel beside the sink.

I went back to bed.

Paul had found sleep. I could hear it in his breathing. I lay down beside him — hip, then shoulder, then adjusting. I had learned to do this without waking him.

His hand found my arm in his sleep. It was the unconscious reach of a man who knew where I was, even when his mind had gone somewhere else for the night.

I closed my eyes.

The water was safe.

Someone had made sure.

CHAPTER 73

Monday, December 7

Paul called from the other room. He needed his reading glasses, which were on the kitchen counter, which I had set there an hour ago when I cleared his breakfast things because he had left them next to his plate again. He knew they were on the counter. He had watched me put them there. He was calling because calling was easier than getting up.

I was sorting the medication.

The weekly organizers were on the counter in front of me, each day's compartment open and waiting.

Paul's blood pressure pill was new as of September. His supplements were arranged in a separate row. Mine were lined up beside his pills. There was a row of supplements we shared by accident of overlapping human chemistry.

"Joy."

"I heard you," I said.

The thing about the medications was that they required attention. Not complicated attention — not the attention of a surgeon — but the attention of counting small things with hands that did not always cooperate, which meant the attention had to compensate for the hands. I had to be present enough to catch a count that the tremor might disrupt. I had been doing this for years. Now I did it for Paul.

He called again.

I set down the bottle I was holding.

Not carefully.

It was not a violent gesture. The bottle did not fall. The pills did not scatter across the counter. I set it down the way you set something down when what you want to do and what you do are in conversation with each other, and what you do wins by a narrow margin.

I stood at the counter and did not reach for his glasses.

From the other room, I could hear the television. It was a game show. Before he retired, he would not have watched it during the day and would have found the noise intrusive. He would have had opinions about wasting time watching such things. Paul watched it now because it was there and the levodopa made him tired in the afternoons, and tired Paul watched things that moved in bright colors and made predictable sounds. I understood this. I had read about it. I had found a study and read it and filed it and explained it to myself at two in the morning when I was awake and he was asleep, and the television was finally off.

Understanding a thing did not make it a thing.

The medication organizer was in front of me. Seven days, two rows, his and mine side by side the way we had been side by side for twenty years, which was either romantic or the universe being creative again — I had not decided. The morning pills and the evening pills, and the as-needed pills would be in their assigned separate cases.

The system. Paul designed it for me. Now I'm sorting the pills for him.

There was a moment — a clear, fully conscious moment — where I considered picking up the organizers and throwing them. I had one in my hand. *Just throw it into the trash.* But it was just a passing thought.

"Joy."

His voice from the other room sounded smaller. Underneath his calling my name was: I need something and I don't want to need it, and I know you are tired, but I don't think I can bring myself to do it.

I knew that. I knew it completely.

I was furious anyway.

Not at Paul. I was furious about the future.

I could see it from here...enough to know that on the counter in front of me, the rows of pills, was a map of something that was going to require more of me than I currently had.

I knew I was going to find the energy required anyway, because that was what you did, when the alternative was not actually an alternative.

But I was allowed to be furious about it. I set the organizer down. I stood there for a moment.

I had been thinking about Rock Steady Boxing for weeks. Rebecca said it gave her more energy...more stamina.

No more thinking about it.

I'll call. Right after I get Paul his glasses…and finish sorting these damned pills.

Then I picked up Paul's glasses from the counter.

Walked to the other room.

He was in his chair, still watching a show. He looked up when I came in, and in his face was the expression of a man who knew he had been waiting longer than the request warranted and had been deciding whether to say so.

I held out his glasses.

"You know," I said, "most people use their legs for this."

He looked at me. His expression shifted — not quite a smile yet, testing the air.

"My legs were busy," he said.

"Doing what, exactly?"

"Holding me in this chair so I didn't fall on my face getting my own glasses."

"That is," I said, "genuinely the best excuse you've ever given me."

He took the glasses. Put them on.

"Thank you," he said.

"You're welcome. I'm going to Rock Steady."

He nodded once. The contestant guessed the last letter. The wheel spun. The room filled with the bright, synthetic sound of something won.

CHAPTER 74

Tuesday, December 8

Paul did not want to come. He had said so...the way he said things he had already decided: not as an argument, not as a request for negotiation, but as a statement of fact delivered to the kitchen in general while looking at his coffee. He didn't feel like going downtown after the support group meeting. The implication, unspoken but present, was that he didn't feel like doing much of anything.

I said, "Come, anyway."

He looked at me over his Styrofoam cup of coffee with the expression he used when he was deciding whether to apply his considerable reasoning abilities to the project of disagreeing with me.

"Fine," he said.

Fine from Paul was the door opening a crack. I had learned to take the crack.

We parked on Main Street and started walking.

Paul walked beside me, holding my hand.

A couple passed us going the other direction, moving fast, the woman talking and the man nodding with the expression of a man who was listening and tracking something on the sidewalk ahead and thinking about something else entirely.

Ordinary people move through their ordinary day without any awareness that they are living wonderfully.

I noticed the first look about a block into our walk.

A man came out of the hardware store, late fifties, holding a paper bag, glanced at Paul and then at me and then wrinkled his forehead— briefly, involuntarily, in the way of a person who has not yet learned to not do this. Not pity exactly. More reflexive than pity.

I had seen this expression before. I knew the look, the way I knew the levodopa cycle, with its afternoon exhaustion and the quality of Paul's stillness when he was searching for a word. It was part of the vocabulary of being visible.

Paul had not seen it. Or had seen it and not registered it. Or had registered it and filed it in the place where he filed things he was not yet ready to look at directly. I did not know which. I decided not to ask.

We walked past the bakery, which smelled of something that had no right being that good.

An older woman coming toward us slowed as she approached, her eyes moving from my hands to Paul's hand. She was perhaps seventy, well-dressed, with the expression of someone who had decided to be helpful before she had decided what help was needed.

"Oh, honey," she said to Paul. "God bless you."

Paul stopped.

I watched him process this. He looked at the woman. He looked at his hand. He looked at the woman again with the expression of a man who was genuinely uncertain whether he had missed something.

"Thank you," he said, because he was Paul and Paul was unfailingly polite even when, perhaps especially when, he had no idea what was happening.

The woman patted his arm — patted it, with the warm finality of a benediction.

Paul watched her go.

"What," he said, "just happened."

"You got blessed," I said.

"I wasn't aware I needed blessing."

"Paul. Look at us. Out here. Tremoring heroically in the cold and you're taking care of a wife who is shaking worse than you. You're basically a Christmas special."

He turned and looked at me.

I kept my face entirely serious.

"A Christmas special," he said.

"Heartwarming. Inspirational. Probably a dog somewhere in the story."

"We don't have a dog."

"The network provides one. For the close-up."

He laughed.

A woman passing by looked over at us. The look was probably just a reflex — looking at two people, one laughing harder than whatever the situation seemed to warrant. Her expression was the familiar one, the half-second of relief, the involuntary gratitude of a person confirming that the thing happening to us was not happening to her.

Paul saw this one. I watched him see it — the laugh still in him, the woman's face registering, the slight shift as he understood what he was looking at.

He looked at me.

I looked back.

"She's relieved," he said laughing even harder.

"Yes. Or wonders if we're both drunks."

"On a Tuesday morning." He laughed in spurts and fits as we started walking again.

When he regained his composure he said, "Does it bother you?"

I considered this honestly. "Sometimes. But I think we're doing them a favor, really. Free existential exercise."

Paul considered this.

"I am not," he said, "a public service."

"You are, though. Think about it. How many people have walked past us this morning and been reminded to call their doctor? To appreciate their steady hands? To hug someone?" I looked at him. "We're basically a wellness campaign. We should charge."

"What would we charge," he said smiling at the thought.

"Sliding scale. The relief look is five dollars. The God bless you...ten. Active pity, we're talking twenty minimum." I paused. "That woman back there? She was relieved and guilty about it. That's a combo. Fifteen."

Paul laughed again. This was the laugh of a man who had found something he had not been looking for and was not sure what to do with it yet but was not putting it down.

We walked.

A teenager coming toward us on the sidewalk looked at us with the expression of someone who did not yet know how to look at illness without staring and had not yet learned that staring was a thing you could choose not to do. He stared. Paul saw him staring. The teenager realized he was staring and looked away with the terrible conspicuousness of someone trying not to be caught doing exactly what he had just been caught doing.

Paul watched him go.

"Five dollars," he said.

"That was the relief look," he said. "Five dollars."

"That was the stare," I said. "The stare is three. He's young. Developing rate card."

"We need a consistent pricing structure."

"We need a laminated menu."

"I'll make one," he said. "This week."

Reaching the corner, we turned and headed back toward the car.

Paul was quiet for half a block.

"I've been thinking about Rock Steady," he said.

"Okay," I said. "Good."

"For the record," Paul said, "I resent being a wellness campaign."

"Noted. I'll put it in the minutes."

"We don't have minutes."

"We should."

He looked sideways at me.

"You're impossible," he said.

"I know," I said. "Five dollars."

He was still smiling when we got to the car.

CHAPTER 75

Wednesday, December 9

Paul had been in the kitchen since four o'clock.

I knew this because the smell arrived in the bedroom before he did — not wrong, just present in the way smells were present when something had been cooking long enough to move through the house and find you wherever you were.

I tried to identify it.

Garlic, yes. Something underneath it — tomato, maybe, or something close to tomato. Something sweet smelling. And onion. Yes, that's it. Onion.

It was a complicated smell. It had layers.

I got up and went to the kitchen, still in my pajamas.

He was at the stove with his back to me, stirring something in the heavy pot we used for soups and the occasional ambitious project. The pot came with us from the apartment on Caldwell Street. Before that, it had lived in Paul's graduate school kitchen. It was the oldest thing in our house. Paul treated it with the reverence of a man who respected things that lasted.

"You're up," he said without turning around.

"I smelled it."

"Good," he stirred. "That means it's working."

I poured coffee, added cream from the refrigerator and then stood at the counter. The set of Paul's shoulders spoke of concentration — not the stressed concentration, the absorbed kind, the kind he had when he was inside something that interested him. He had been moving through the house for two weeks with the depleted quality of someone running on the wrong fuel. This was different. This was Paul with a project.

"What is it?" I asked.

"Ragu," he said it with the slight elevation of a man who had been looking forward to saying it. "Not from the jar. The actual thing. Low and slow."

"You've been up since four."

"The onion needed time."

I laughed.

"I found a recipe. An old one. From a cooking magazine." He paused. "The one from the box."

He tasted his ragu, "She dog-eared the page," he said as he stirred. "I thought that meant something."

CHAPTER 76

Wednesday, December 9

We ate at six-thirty because that was when Paul said his sauce was ready, which was when he had planned for it to be ready.

He set the table: placemats, forks, the good bowls. He even put a candle in the center of the table and lit it.

He brought the pot to the table.

The smell came up with the steam.

The garlic was still there. The tomato was still there. But alongside them there was something I couldn't name. It arrived with the steam and sat at the back of my throat.

Not spoiled. Not wrong in any way I could point to. Just — wrong for me. Wrong in the way things sometimes smelled wrong. I had no explanation for it, but I couldn't argue with it.

Paul ladled noodles and ragu into my bowl.

The smell intensified with the closeness.

I picked up my fork.

I put it down.

Paul was ladling his own bowl. He set the pot back, replaced the lid, and sat down.

He picked up his fork.

He took a bite.

His face showed his plan had worked — he smiled and nodded like a man accounting for his victories.

"Well," he said. He looked at me.

My fork was beside my bowl. I had my hands in my lap.

He looked at my bowl.

"It smells wrong," I said.

The words arrived before I decided to say them. I didn't say the managed version — *I'm not very hungry*, or *I had something earlier,* the small fictions I had been placing between myself and the true thing for four years. Just: "it smells wrong."

He set his fork down.

I looked at my bowl. "It's Parkinson's."

I said, "I can't tell you what it smells like. It just isn't...right."

"You got up at four," I said. "You used her recipe. I'm sorry. Maybe later I'll try again."

Paul frowned. "Is it all of it? Or just the garlic?"

"I don't know." I picked up my fork and brought it close to the bowl, trying to isolate what was arriving. "The garlic. And something underneath." I set the fork down. "I'm sorry."

"Don't apologize for it." He said it without sharpness. "It's not yours to apologize for."

"Eat yours," I said.

"I'm not particularly—"

“Paul. Eat it. You made it. I can tell it's good. The wrongness isn't in the food.”

He picked up his fork.

I watched him eat and thought about my mother folding the corner of a page, the quality of her dog-ears, which were never casual — she folded corners with intention, which meant she had made this or intended to make this or had given it to someone she thought would make it. I didn’t know which. The magazine had been in the box with the other things she hadn't gotten around to sorting.

“She would have been pleased,” I said. “That you used it.”

He took another bite.

“I'll find something else,” I said. “For dinner.”

“The crackers are in the third cabinet.”

“I know where the crackers are.” I opened the cupboard door.

“That's the thing,” I said. “Isn't it?”

He looked at me.

“You can do everything right,” I said. “Something in me has changed.” I held his gaze.

I got the crackers from the third cabinet and brought them to the table and sat back down across from him. We ate our separate dinners in the kitchen where the ragu smell was still present and wrong for me and right for the room. Neither of us said anything for a while.

After a moment, I reached across and tore a piece of bread from the loaf beside the pot, and I held it close. The bread smelled like bread, clean and plain and entirely what it was.

I ate the chunk of bread.

"Better?" Paul asked.

"Yes."

"I'll make bread next time."

"You don't have to make anything next time."

"I know I don't have to. Tell me something," he said.

"What kind of something?"

"Anything." He looked at the table. "Something I don't know."

"My mother burned things constantly," I said. "She was a terrible judge of heat. She'd get interested in something else and forget to watch." I looked at the bread in my hands. "She burned soup once." I paused. "She served it anyway. Said the char gave it character."

"Did it?"

"No," I said. "It was terrible. But we ate it. I kept wishing my mother would leave the kitchen, so I could dump my bowl."

"She sounds like she was difficult," he said. "Tell me more."

So, I did.

CHAPTER 77

Tuesday, December 15

We ended up at the cafe. Not by plan — Rebecca and I had walked out of the community center and turned in the same direction without discussing it, and by the time we had walked two blocks, it was obvious where we were going.

Inside, the familiar smell greeted us. The woman in yellow wasn't there. A young man, a college student by the look of him, led us to a booth without asking if we had a preference. He had sized us up at the door and arrived at the conclusion: a booth by the window.

The vinyl squeaked when we sat down.

We looked at each other.

"Same table," Rebecca said.

I nodded.

"The eggs are still reliable," Rebecca said. "In case you'd forgotten."

"It's only been a few days."

"One day to many," she said.

She added, "The coffee remains a federal offense."

I closed the menu. "I'll have the coffee."

"Of course you will."

The college student came back. We ordered the same things we had ordered the first time. He wrote it down with the slightly aggrieved efficiency of someone who considered this work a temporary arrangement, which it probably was, and went away.

"Steve opened the journal," she said.

"Oh?"

"Not to read it. He opened the packaging. Set it on my nightstand with a pen beside it. He didn't say anything about it."

"How long ago?"

"Three weeks."

"Have you written in it?"

She looked out of the window. "No."

The coffee arrived in the heavy white mugs. I wrapped both hands around mine. The ceramic was warm and satisfying.

"I started typing instead," Rebecca said.

I thought about the dictation software. My voice in the empty kitchen, the microphone catching what my hands had stopped being able to catch. Eleanor's words in my mouth because they had stopped coming reliably from my fingers. The quality of the sentences when I spoke sounded different from what I would have written, looser in some places and more precise in others. *The voice is a different instrument.*

"I'm still writing, dictating" I said.

Something shifted in her face — like she had heard confirmation.

"The novel," she said.

"Yes. I thought dictating would feel like losing something. But speaking it, the sentences come out differently. Sometimes better. Like my voice knows things the fingers have to work up to."

"I probably won't write in the journal," she said, "I hate when Steve's right. He takes it very quietly, which is somehow worse."

We ate our food.

Before we got up from the table I said, "I signed up Friday. I'm going on Thursday," I said.

"Good."

CHAPTER 78

Wednesday, December 16

The newspaper was in front of him, still folded. The coffee maker had finished. His mug was on the hook. He was looking at the middle distance over the newspaper with the expression he had when he was thinking about something he had not yet given himself permission to say.

I poured my coffee. Stood at the counter for a moment, watching him not read. Then I filled his cup.

"Sections are in order," I said.

He looked up. "What?"

"The newspaper."

I went to the table. "You haven't opened it."

He looked at the paper as if noticing it for the first time. "I was going to."

"You've been sitting here twenty minutes."

Paul reached for his mug, hit the edge of mine, caught it before my coffee went all the way over. It wasn't dramatic. Just enough so that coffee drizzled down my cup onto the paper. But then his hand bumped into his own cup. This resulted in a somewhat larger pool that spread across the newspaper before either of us moved. Spread through the sports section first.

Then, without deciding to, he reached for my mug.

He was trying to pull it back from the spreading edge. His right hand closed around it and the tremor was in him and my mug went over.

The sound it made was not loud. Ceramic on the table, the mug on its side, my coffee moving to meet his. The two of them finding each other across the ruined newspaper, mixing, dark and spreading, running off the table's edge onto the chair and the floor.

Paul's hand was still where the mug had been.

I didn't move. "Paul."

He didn't answer immediately. "I had a plan," he said.

"Which plan."

"Before. When I thought it was just stress. I had a plan for us. After your diagnosis, I had a revised plan."

"I know," I said.

"There aren't enough columns," he said, "for what's happening."

The mug was on its side. The newspaper was ruined.

He looked at the table. The mess of it. Coffee spreading in both directions from the wreckage of his two attempts to manage it.

"I don't know how to be inside it."

The coffee had stopped moving.

"You came downtown," I said.

He looked at me.

"You didn't want to come. You came anyway. You laughed at a stranger's blessing on a public sidewalk, and you invented a pricing structure for other people's discomfort, and then you told me you'd been thinking about Rock Steady." I held his gaze. "That's not outside it."

"That's what being inside it looks like," I said. "It's not a plan."

I said, "Tomorrow I'm going. I don't know what's going to happen. I don't know if I can do any of it. I have no columns for it."

He looked at the mess.

"I'm afraid," he said. "Of tomorrow. Not the way I've been afraid of everything since Little Rock. This is — I'm afraid you're going to find something there that I can't give you. Some room where you can be someone, I won't know how to help you be."

"Paul."

He looked up.

"I wrecked your coffee," he said.

"And the sports section."

Picking up Paul's cup, I made an impulsive decision and turned it over.

As the last of his coffee ran out, I said, "That's better. The whole paper."

"It was yesterday's anyway." He smiled. "The Thompson kid. The pitcher. He got the scholarship."

"I know. You told me."

"He's starting in the spring. I thought about going to watch him pitch." He paused. "I thought maybe you'd like to go."

"To a baseball game?"

"Just the one." He said it with something careful and fragile underneath it, the voice of a man who had just promised himself something. "If the weather's decent. If we feel like it."

I stood and got the dish towel.

Paul looked at the towel.

"In a minute," I said sitting down.

He nodded.

"The spring," I said.

"If the weather's decent."

He looked at the dish towel sitting on the table doing nothing.

The laugh came out of him quietly. Not the Main Street laugh — smaller, more private. The laugh of a man alone with his wife in his own kitchen, with cold coffee on the floor and a ruined newspaper and a dish towel placed with ceremony beside the problem it was meant to solve.

I started laughing too.

Then I picked up the dish towel, and we cleaned up our mess together.

CHAPTER 79

Thursday, December 17

Thursday came the way things came when you had stopped trying to hurry them — quietly, without announcement.

Paul was in the kitchen when I came down. Coffee already made. He looked up, and we looked at each other across the kitchen. There was nothing to say that hadn't already been said, so neither of us said anything. I poured coffee and drank it black, managed to drink half of it. I drank it while standing at the counter the way I used to drink coffee in the mornings when I was going to work.

"Drive safe," he said. "My intake session is this evening. I won't be far behind you."

I nodded.

The wind chime hanging beside the door reminded me of my purpose. I touched it — and went out.

CHAPTER 80

Thursday, December 17

The drive was ten minutes. I turned into the parking lot.

I am here now. The engine is off and the building is in front of me and in a moment, I will open the door and walk across the parking lot and that will be the beginning of the next thing.

I opened the door.

CHAPTER 81

Thursday, December 17

The gym smelled of rubber and effort and the institutional cleanliness of a space run by a hospital — the cleanliness of somewhere that took the body seriously, that believed the body was worth the equipment and the space and the careful maintenance of both. It was not a beautiful gym. High ceilings, industrial lighting, rows of equipment in the middle of a large space.

In one room, someone had set out chairs in a circle. People were beginning to find them.

I stood in the doorway for a moment. Not hesitating — arriving, taking in the room.

The first thing I noticed and the thing that mattered most was the normalcy of the room, despite its purpose. Everyone seemed comfortable with who they were and where we were.

A man with a walker, moved with the deliberateness of someone who had negotiated this territory many times. A woman already seated, smiled at me.

And then I saw Rebecca. She waved me over to the seat beside her.

I was sitting down when I saw Gerald walk in. He had clearly been here before. The way he interacted with everyone was more open than the way he held himself at the support group meetings. He had not mentioned going to Rock Steady. That was so entirely Gerald that something loosened in my chest that I hadn't known was tight.

Across the circle I found Tara. She was talking quietly to one of the assistant coaches. Taking her seat, she met my eyes across the circle.

A volunteer moved through the space carrying her water bottle, checking in with people, with the easy familiarity of someone who had been doing this long enough to know which faces were new and who needed what.

The coach was a woman, whose physical appearance spoke of someone who had spent years taking care of herself. Her presence exuded respect for everyone in the room. I imagined she had spent years thinking about what bodies could do, if they were encouraged and trusted to do it. She looked around the circle, and the room settled.

She said, "I want to tell you why we introduce ourselves before we start. Because it matters."

Another person came in and sat down.

"Parkinson's takes a lot of things," the coach said. "One of the things it works on is the voice. Softens it. Parkinson's wants to shrink you."

She looked around the circle. "It works on how large you let yourself be in a room. Some of you know what I mean. You start making yourself smaller. Taking up less space. Disappearing a little at a time."

I knew exactly what she was referring to.

"We say our names out loud, at full voice, in this room, every single session, because your name tells us who you are. Who you are is one thing the disease does not get to have."

She took a moment to look at each person in the circle.

The coach said, "Saying your name here is a refusal to disappear…We'll go around. When you say your name, say it like you're not small...you're a fighter...fighting for your life... for your right to be you."

The introductions moved around the circle.

The introductions moved closer.

It was my turn.

I didn't hesitate.

"Hello Rock Steady. My name is Joy."

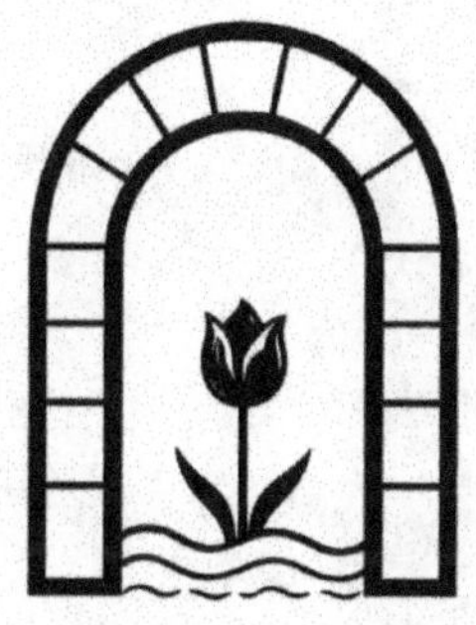

LIMINAL GROUND

LITERARY PRESS

About the Author

J.D. Roff is a writer, artist, and scholar living with early-onset Parkinson's disease. Roff holds a master's degree in Consciousness Studies. A former preacher and spiritual teacher, Roff enjoys exploring Scripture, the intersection of mysticism, esoteric history, and the nature of the self. Roff's research has been published in more than thirty books under a pen name.

Spilled Coffee is Roff's first published novel.

Roff knows what it costs to stay present in a life that is changing faster than you can manage it. That knowledge is on every page.

www.ingramcontent.com/pod-product-compliance
Lightning Source LLC
LaVergne TN
LVHW010636110826
845149LV00014B/2850
* 9 7 8 1 9 7 2 5 2 0 0 1 7 *